THE

LOW-FODMAP

COOKBOOK

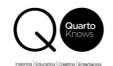

Brimming with creative inspiration, how-to projects, and useful information to enrich your everyday life, Quarto Knows is a favorite destination for those pursuing their interests and passions. Visit our site and dig deeper with our books into your area of interest: Quarto Creates, Quarto Cooks, Quarto Homes, Quarto Lives, Quarto Drives, Quarto Explores, Quarto Gifts, or Quarto Kids.

First published in 2016 by Fair Winds Press,
an imprint of The Quarto Group,
100 Cummings Center, Suite 265-D,
Beverly, MA 01915, USA.
T (978) 282-9590 F (978) 283-2742
www.QuartoKnows.com

Fair Winds Press titles are also available at discount for retail, wholesale, promotional, and bulk purchase. For details, contact the Special Sales Manager by email at specialsales@quarto.com or by mail at The Quarto Group, Attn: Special Sales Manager, 401 Second Avenue North, Suite 310, Minneapolis, MN 55401, USA.

20 19 18   6

ISBN: 978-1-59233-714-9

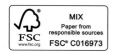

Digital edition published in 2016
eISBN: 978-1-63159-161-7

Library of Congress Cataloging-in-Publication Data

Names: Benjamin, Dianne, 1952- author.
Title: The low-FODMAP cookbook : 100 delicious, gut-friendly recipes for IBS
    and other digestive disorders / Dianne Fastenow Benjamin.
Other titles: Low-Fermentable Oligosaccharides, Disaccharides,
    Monosaccharides and Polyols cookbook
Description: Beverly, Massachusetts : Fair Winds Press, 2016.
Identifiers: LCCN 2016003826 (print) | LCCN 2016009947 (ebook) | ISBN
    9781592337149 (paperback) | ISBN 9781631591617 ()
Subjects: LCSH: Malabsorption syndromes--Diet therapy--Recipes. | Irritable
    colon--Diet therapy--Recipes. | BISAC: COOKING / Health & Healing /
    General. | HEALTH & FITNESS / Diseases / Abdominal. | LCGFT: Cookbooks.
Classification: LCC RC862.M3 B35 2016 (print) | LCC RC862.M3 (ebook) | DDC
    641.5/631--dc23
LC record available at http://lccn.loc.gov/2016003826

Cover and Book Design: Megan Jones Design
Page Layout: Megan Jones Design
Photography: Dianne Fastenow Benjamin except images by Shutterstock (p. 9, 79, 107, and 142)

Printed in China

The information in this book is for educational purposes only. It is not intended to replace the advice of a physician or medical practitioner. Please see your health-care provider before beginning any new health program.

THE
LOW-FODMAP
COOKBOOK

100 Delicious, Gut-Friendly Recipes
for IBS and other Digestive Disorders

DIANNE FASTENOW BENJAMIN

FAIR WINDS

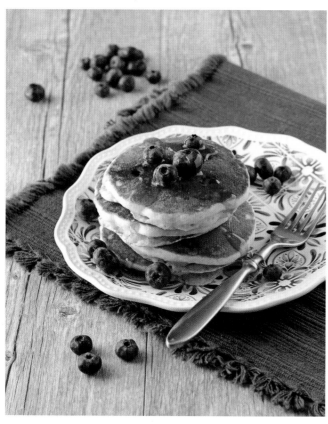
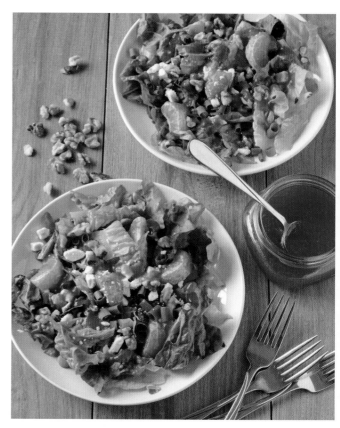
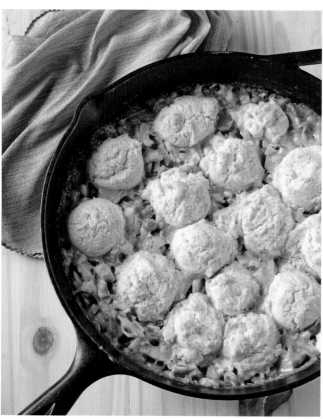
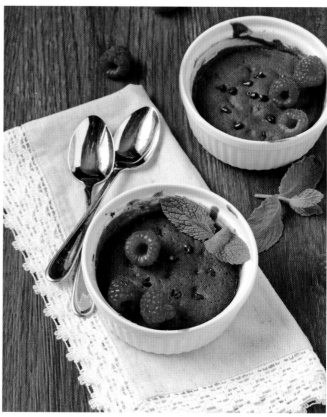

CONTENTS

INTRODUCTION

My passion for food began when I was about eight or nine years old. I had a *Better Homes and Gardens* kids' cookbook that I loved: My mom taught me how to follow the recipes, and my friends and I baked and baked—and baked some more. I've got vivid memories of making treats like snickerdoodles, yellow cake with chocolate frosting, and caramel corn. (That caramel corn was so good that my dad still talks about it to this day!)

We don't have any chefs or restaurateurs in our family—unless you count my great-great-grandfather, who was a baker—but food has always been a big part of our lives. After my husband and I got married, we noticed a major difference in our respective families. When we get together with his family, the question on everyone's lips is, "What are we *doing* today?" But when we get together with *my* family, everyone asks, "What are we *eating* today?" Food is truly the main event: Vacations, holidays, and birthdays are always centered around where—and what—we're going to eat. So it's no surprise that I've been collecting and creating recipes almost obsessively since I was a teenager or that I love to share recipes that I've tried and created on my blog, Delicious as it Looks (www.deliciousasitlooks.com). I started Delicious as it Looks in 2010, after I discovered my talent for photographing food. I was still eating like an average person back then; but while I tried to eat as healthfully and naturally as possible, my digestive system was a mess.

I was diagnosed with irritable bowel syndrome (IBS) almost twenty years ago. Symptoms would come and go: Sometimes I'd feel okay, but the rest of the time I felt like there was something seriously wrong with me. Finally, after all my tests came back normal, I got the IBS diagnosis. I continued to suffer until I finally took matters into my own hands and began researching how diet affects IBS. That was nothing new for me: I've been interested in health and nutrition since I lost fifty pounds as a teenager by counting calories, exercising, and using diet tips gleaned from women's magazines, so taking the initiative and researching diets and digestive issues felt like a natural extension of that curiosity.

At last I landed on the low-FODMAP diet, which completely changed my life. Suddenly, everything made sense. The foods I was eating were actually causing my symptoms! It was a revelation at the time, but looking back, it seems so obvious. So why did I have to figure this out all by myself? The answer is simple: I was diagnosed before anyone had even heard of FODMAPs. And that means I missed out. (These days, I hope IBS sufferers will learn about FODMAPs from their doctors when they're diagnosed.)

And, of course, adopting a low-FODMAP diet posed a challenge for my blog. "Now what?" I thought. "I can't eat *anything*!" But it wasn't long before I made the decision to stay positive and to focus on all of the foods I *can* eat. After that, I started developing recipes that use low-FODMAP ingredients and sharing them on my blog. If you look through my blog's archives, you'll see how I transitioned from a "normal" diet to a low-FODMAP one (and how I dabbled in a grain-free diet for a while en route). It's been such an interesting and enjoyable experience, and the best part is that my experience—and my recipes—have helped so many people.

It's my hope that this book will help you, too. It will show you how to make 100 low-FODMAP recipes, everything from hearty stews to healthy pasta dishes to decadent chocolate chip cookies. I'm confident it will prove that eating low-FODMAP is anything but boring! Also, as you'll see, lots of these recipes can easily be made vegan with just a couple of simple substitutions and many of them are gluten-free, too.

Let's get started!

—Dianne Fastenow Benjamin

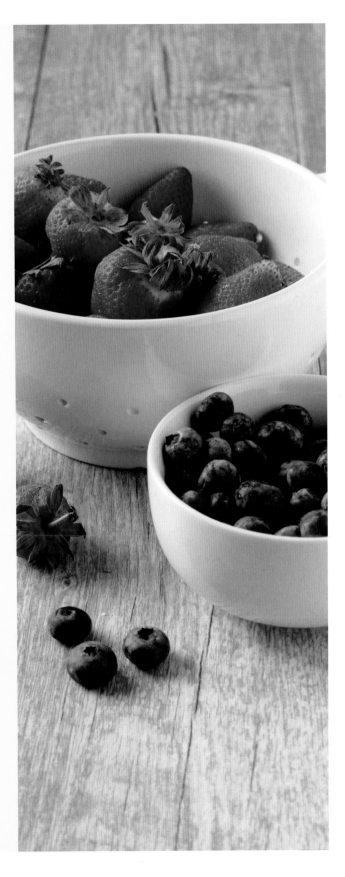

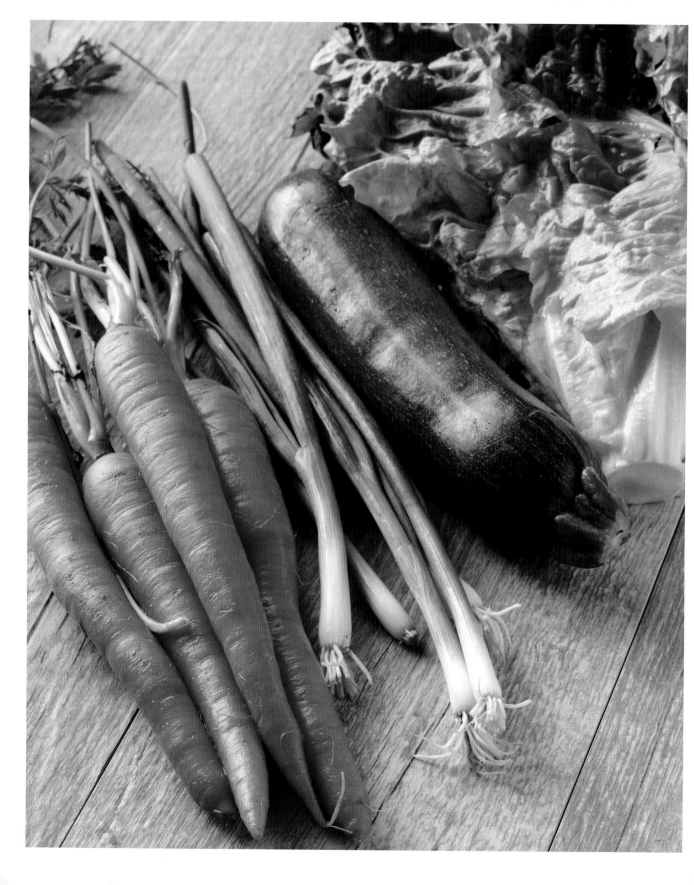

FODMAPS AND THE LOW-FODMAP DIET

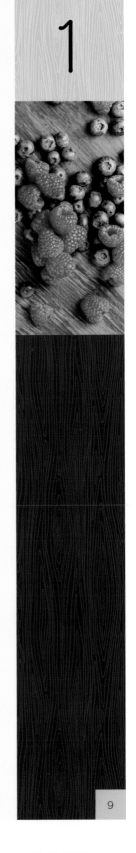

Irritable bowel syndrome (IBS) affects about 20 percent of adults in the United States, and recent research shows that enjoying a low-FODMAP diet can help drastically reduce your IBS symptoms. But what are FODMAPs, and what do they mean for your digestive system? It's a fairly complicated subject, but I will break it down for you so that will have an understanding of the following:

- What FODMAPs are

- What common foods contain FODMAPs

- Why FODMAPs cause digestive issues in some people

- How the diet works, including the elimination and rechallenge phases

- The difference between a food intolerance and a food allergy

- How to improve your digestion

- What foods to enjoy on the low-FODMAP diet

"FODMAP" stands for "Fermentable, Oligosaccharides, Disaccharides, Monosaccharides, And Polyols." These are carbohydrates (or sugars) that are poorly absorbed in the small intestine. They end up traveling to the large intestine, where they become the perfect food for the bacteria that live in the large intestine. The bacteria eat away at these sugars and cause fermentation, which results in nasty symptoms like gas, pain, cramping, diarrhea, constipation, and nausea—typical symptoms for people who suffer from IBS. Being small molecules, they also attract water into the small intestine, causing symptoms. The term *FODMAPs* has been coined relatively recently, and it's getting a lot of press in the diet and nutrition world these days since some people who thought they were sensitive to dietary gluten have realized that they're actually suffering from a sensitivity to the fructans, or sugars, in wheat.

Research from Monash University in Melbourne, Australia, shows that avoiding FODMAPs can greatly improve symptoms in up to 76 percent of IBS patients.

Before we launch into the details of the low-FODMAP diet, let's start with a brief refresher course in nutrition. The food we eat consists of three components: carbohydrates, proteins, and fats. Some foods consist mostly of protein (like the extra-lean ground turkey in tacos) and some foods consist of fat (like the olive oil you drizzle on salads). Other foods are completely carbohydrate-based, like the sugar you sprinkle on your morning oatmeal. And in terms of a low-FODMAP diet, the component we're most concerned about is carbohydrates.

Carbohydrates, which consist of sugars, starches, and fiber, are an important component of our diets since they provide our bodies with energy. Here's how: Our digestive systems break down the carbs we eat until they can be absorbed through the intestinal wall into the bloodstream, where they're converted into energy. And they're in a lot of the foods we eat, including fruits, vegetables, breads, and pasta. But certain carbs—the FODMAPs—can cause issues in people with IBS and other digestive disorders.

Carbohydrates include monosaccharides (such as glucose, fructose, and galactose); disaccharides (for example sucrose—composed of glucose and fructose and lactose—composed of glucose and galactose); polyols (such as sorbitol and mannitol); oligosaccharides (such as fructooligosaccharides and galactooligsaccharides), and polysaccharides (resistant starch and non-starch polysaccharides, also known as fiber).

Starches come from plant-based foods, like grains, vegetables, and fruit. When you eat starchy foods, natural enzymes in your digestive system break the starch down into the simplest sugars—glucose, fructose, and galactose—which are then absorbed into the bloodstream. But some carbohydrates (known as FODMAPs) are poorly absorbed in the small intestine. While malabsorption of these carbohydrates is a normal event (for example, the human intestine lacks enzymes to digest oligosaccharides and approximately 40% of the population regardless of an IBS diagnosis malabsorbs fructose); it is the response to this malabsorption that is abnormal in people with IBS. In people with IBS, the bowel wall is hypersensitive to stimulation (visceral hypersensitivity) and is more likely to cause pain when stimulated. Therefore, when FODMAP containing foods are consumed, there is an influx of water and gas into the intestines, causing stretching and distension. In the presence of visceral hypersensitivity, this stretching and distension may induce symptoms of pain, bloating, abdominal distension, diarrhea, and/or constipation.

Now that you've gotten a quick rundown on what carbs are and how they're digested, here's a brief overview of each FODMAP carbohydrate and the foods in which they occur. We already know that the **F** in **FODMAP** stands for **"fermentable."** Fermentation happens when intestinal bacteria consume the undigested carbohydrates in the large intestine, creating gas.

Oligosaccharides are chains of sugars, such as:

- **Fructans** (or fructooligosaccharides)—Fructans are chains of fructose molecules. They are found in onions, garlic, wheat, chicory root (inulin), asparagus, and artichokes.

- **GOS** (also known as galacto-oligosaccharides) —GOS are polymers of galactose, glucose, and fructose. They are found in beans, legumes, peas, and soybeans.

Disaccharides are two monosaccharides linked together, such as:

- **Lactose**—Lactose is composed of one glucose and one galactose molecule and is found in dairy products such as milk and soft cheeses. Lactose only causes trouble for the small minority of folks who lack the enzyme that's necessary for breaking it down.

Monosaccharides contain only a single sugar molecule, such as:

- **Fructose**—Fructose is found in fruits and sweeteners. From a low-FODMAP perspective, we're only concerned with the fruits that contain an *excess* of fructose—that is, more fructose than glucose. That doesn't apply to all fruits and sweeteners. For example, sucrose (granulated sugar) is composed of one fructose molecule and one glucose molecule. Because the glucose helps the body to absorb the fructose, granulated sugar is well tolerated

F ermentable
+
O ligosaccharides
+
D isaccharides
+
M onosaccharides
+
A nd
+
P olyols
- - - - - - - - - - - - - - - - - -
= **FODMAP!**

by folks with IBS. Foods that contain more fructose than glucose (excess of fructose), like apples, pears, mangoes, honey, high-fructose corn syrup (HFCS), and agave nectar should be avoided.

Polyols are sugar alcohols, such as:

- **Xylitol**, **mannitol**, **sorbitol**, and **maltitol**— These are naturally found in mushrooms, apples, and stone fruits (such as peaches, nectarines, apricots, plums, and cherries). They're also found in processed foods such as sugar-free sweeteners, which turn up in sugar-free chewing gum and candy.

How the Low-FODMAP Diet Can Help

The low-FODMAP diet shows you how to figure out which foods are your personal "triggers," and then it helps you avoid those foods in order to manage your IBS symptoms. The diet is generally divided into two phases. First is the elimination phase, in which you eliminate high-FODMAP foods from your diet for two to six weeks. The second phase is the reintroduction phase, or "rechallenge" phase. In this stage, you'll intentionally eat higher-FODMAP foods in order to test your reactions to them. After that, it's up to you to avoid the foods that cause your symptoms.

Before we go any further, let's talk about what the low-FODMAP diet is *not*. Although it has the word "diet" in its name, **the low-FODMAP diet is not intended for weight loss**. Also, it isn't black and white. Notice that it's called a *low*-FODMAP diet and not a FODMAP-*free* diet? That's because it's nearly impossible to eat absolutely zero FODMAPs and still maintain a healthy diet. Unless all you eat is meat—and that's hardly a balanced eating plan!—you're going to end up eating *some* FODMAPs. The trick is to minimize them to the point at which your symptoms improve. And it's important to not be too restrictive in the process, or you could end up suffering from malnutrition.

The low-FODMAP diet is not necessarily a gluten-free diet. Gluten is a *protein* found in wheat, barley, and rye, which celiacs must eliminate from their diets. But wheat, barley, and rye also contain FODMAPs, which are *carbohydrates*. It is possible for people with celiac disease to have IBS-like symptoms as well: These folks should continue to eat gluten-free, but they might want to consider reducing their consumption of FODMAPs, too. While research is currently being conducted on the existence of non-celiac gluten sensitivity, it may actually be the fructans, not the gluten, in wheat that cause reactions in some people. Keep in mind that gluten-free foods are not necessarily low-FODMAP foods. Wheat-free foods may contain high-FODMAP ingredients, such as onions, garlic, or pear juice, to name a few.

The low-FODMAP protocol is not one size fits all. Not everyone reacts to the same foods in the same way. You may find that you can tolerate some FODMAPs—but you may also find that you can't tolerate them at all. Either way, it's good to know, and that's the whole point: The low-FODMAP diet is all about *you* and how *you* react to certain foods.

Ultimately, the low-FODMAP diet is a tool to help you feel your best. So don't panic—this protocol doesn't mean that you'll have to say goodbye to your favorite foods forever! The elimination phase of the diet (usually 2 to 6 weeks in duration) is the most restrictive, but afterward, you'll reintroduce new foods, and ideally you'll find out that you can tolerate more than just the "safe" foods. Plus, food intolerances can change over time, so you might want to wait a few months before testing certain foods again. You may find that you're able to tolerate them the next time around.

Malabsorbed FODMAPs
    +
Fermentation & Osmotic Activity
    +
Hypersensitivity or Bacterial Overgrowth

= IBS

CONSULT A PROFESSIONAL

As you've probably noticed, the low-FODMAP diet is pretty complicated, and putting it into practice usually requires the assistance of a professional. Always consult with a doctor or dietitian before embarking on the strict phase of the low FODMAP diet. She or he can guide you through the process safely, ensuring that your diet remains nutritionally adaquate. A dietitian will also be helpful in the rechallenge phase, in helping you to identify which foods and FODAMPs trigger your symptoms. Visit medical nutrition therapist Patsy Catsos's website, www.ibsfree.net, for a useful list of dietitians around the world who have experience in the low-FODMAP diet. If you can't find one in your area, check out these resources and books, and review them with your doctor:

- *The Monash University Low FODMAP Diet App* for smartphones
- *IBS—Free at Last!* by Patsy Catsos
- *The Complete Low-FODMAP Diet* by Sue Shepherd
- *The Low-FODMAP 28-Day Plan: A Healthy Cookbook with Gut-Friendly Recipes for IBS Relief* by Kate Scarlata

THE ELIMINATION PHASE

I like to think of the low-FODMAP approach as a kind of an experiment that you conduct on your digestive system. As with any scientific experiment, you need a test subject (you!), a control (the low-FODMAP diet), and a variable (high-FODMAP foods). Finally, repeated trials (the challenge phase) are needed to establish a conclusion.

In the first phase, the elimination phase, FODMAPs are avoided as much as possible for four to six weeks. If you don't feel any better after four to six weeks, the low-FODMAP approach may not be for you, and you may want to talk to your doctor about trying a different approach. Remember, most studies show the low FODMAP diet is effective in only around three quarters of people. For everyone else, other factors may trigger symptoms.

Keep these important tips in mind during the elimination phase:

- **Eat a well-balanced diet.** Include foods from each of the food groups—protein, grains, fruits and vegetables, and dairy, if desired—in every meal. When it comes to fruits and vegetables, keep it colorful. The more color in the produce, the more vitamins and nutrients it contains.

- **Stick to the serving sizes recommended by your dietitian or doctor.**

- **Keep the overall FODMAP load low throughout the day.** In other words, if you're going to eat foods that have some FODMAPs (for instance, a little milk in your coffee or a little celery on your salad), don't eat them all at once. Instead, spread them throughout the day. Sue Shepherd, author of *The Complete Low-FODMAP Diet*, recommends eating no more than one serving of fruit at a sitting in order to spread out the fructose load.

- **Keep a food diary.** This will help you keep track of what foods you're eating and of any resulting symptoms.

- **Avoid foods that you already know you're sensitive to.**

- **If you are unsure if a food is low-FODMAP or not, don't eat it until you're in the rechallenge phase.**

THE RECHALLENGE PHASE

During the rechallenge phase, or reintroduction phase, FODMAPs are systematically reintroduced into your diet to see whether they produce symptoms. This phase will take about six weeks to complete, but it's worth it. You'll have identified your trigger foods, and you'll be better able to manage your symptoms. The challenge phase follows these basic steps:

- **Reintroduce one FODMAP at a time.** Try to choose a food that contains only one FODMAP; for example, the fructans in wheat or the lactose in milk.

- **Eat a typical serving of the FODMAP food (such as one slice of bread or half a cup [120 ml] of milk) and record your symptoms over the next 24 hours.** If symptoms occur, then it's likely that that food, eaten in that quantity, is a trigger. If no symptoms are present, then you'll know that it's safe to eat the FODMAP food in that amount.

- **If symptoms do occur, wait for them to abate before you test again.**

- Next, you can either **try a new FODMAP food or retest the same food you tried in step 2, only in a larger or smaller serving.** If you couldn't tolerate the food you tested in its standard serving size, you might try it in a smaller amount (for example, half a slice of bread or a quarter cup [60 ml] of milk). If you were able to tolerate the food you tested, you can try eating more of it (for example, two slices of bread or one cup [235 ml] of milk). In this way, you'll be able to determine your individual threshold for particular foods.

- **Repeat this process until you've tested all the FODMAP foods you want.** Always remember to wait until any symptoms subside before testing again. And try to reintroduce foods that contain only one type of FODMAP at a time; that way, it'll be easier to isolate the FODMAPs that you can—or can't—tolerate.

What if the Low-FODMAP Diet Doesn't Work for Me?

While the low-FODMAP diet has made a world of a difference for me and many of the readers of my blog, this approach will not work for everyone. Like I said earlier, the low-FODMAP diet isn't one size fits all. If you don't notice any improvement after you complete the elimination and challenge phases, you might want to explore other food intolerances or allergies. For example, after a while I realized that I was reacting badly to eggs even though they aren't high in FODMAPs.

The FDA recognizes these eight foods as the most common allergens: milk, eggs, fish, shellfish, tree nuts, peanuts, wheat, and soybeans. According to *Food Allergies and Food Intolerance* by Jonathan Brostoff and Linda Gamlin, commonly reported food intolerances include corn, potatoes, rice, and sesame. These foods rarely provoke a true allergic response, but they can be common culprits when it comes to food intolerance.

OTHER SYMPTOM-CAUSING FOODS

Foods containing FODMAPs have been shown to cause or aggravate IBS symptoms, but some low-FODMAP or FODMAP-free foods seem to be problematic, too. It's a good idea to keep these to a minimum when you're trying to relieve your symptoms:

- **Foods that are high in fat.** Patients with IBS often identify fatty meals as a trigger for IBS symptoms, such as bloating. This may be due to the changes in gut motility (movement of food and fluid through the intestinal tract) that are induced by fat and exaggerated in people with IBS.

- **Spicy foods.** Although red chiles are considered low-FODMAP in limited serving sizes, they're still spicy, and they also contain a substance called capsaicin. A study published in 2008 in *Gut*, the official journal of the British Society of Gastroenterology, indicated that people with IBS may have more capsaicin receptors in the colon, which results in pain and hypersensitivity. People who suspect they are sensitive to spicy foods should avoid them during the elimination diet.

- **Caffeine.** We all know that caffeine is a stimulant, since it does such a good job of waking us up in the morning—but it also stimulates your digestive system. This isn't necessarily a bad thing, but it may cause diarrhea in some people.

- **Alcohol.** People with IBS often identify alcohol as a symptom trigger, however, studies have not confirmed whether removing or reducing alcohol intake improves symptom control.

True allergies can be diagnosed by a skin-prick test, in which a small amount of purified allergen is injected into the skin and then left alone in order to see whether an immune response occurs at the site. A food intolerance is much more difficult to detect and involves—you guessed it!—an elimination diet. However, there is no firm guidance on how to implement an elimination diet, in terms of the foods consumed in the elimination period or the type and quantity of food introduced in the reintroduction period. Elimination diets are also labor intensive and time-consuming to complete and being highly restrictive, they may compromise nutritional status.

Food additives may also prevent the low-FODMAP diet from working for you. For example, my husband and I both recently suspected that we were having bad reactions to xanthan gum, an emulsifier that's commonly added to gluten-free products. This is why none of the recipes in this book call for it. A recent study by the Georgia State University Institute for Biomedical Sciences suggested that there could be a link between emulsifying additives in foods and IBS: Such emulsifiers may disturb gut microbiota, which promotes inflammation and can lead to colitis. However, this was an early study in mice, so data from human studies are needed to confirm these results.

NINE WAYS TO IMPROVE YOUR DIGESTION

These tips are great for boosting digestive health, whether or not you have IBS. But if you're in the challenge phase of the low-FODMAP diet, it's especially important to keep an eye on your digestion since you're potentially putting it under added stress by reintroducing foods that it might have trouble tolerating. That's why it's best to focus on the following:

- **Eat on a schedule.** Eat meals around the same time each day so that your digestive system knows what to expect. This will also keep your body well-fueled throughout the day. Plus, you won't get overly hungry, which can lead to poor food choices.

- **Eat smaller, more frequent meals for optimum digestion.** Don't overload or overwhelm your digestive system.

- **Eat slowly and mindfully.** Take the time to sit down and eat. Remember that digestion starts in the mouth, so focus on chewing your food.

- **Avoid activities that can cause gas**, such as chewing gum, drinking through a straw, and drinking carbonated beverages.

- **Minimize stress.** Our minds and digestive systems are intrinsically linked. If your mind is stressed out, your gut will be, too. Try meditation or exercises such as progressive muscle relaxation or soak in a warm bath.

- **Exercise.** There is no conclusive proof that exercising can improve IBS symptoms, but incorporating exercise into your daily routine is important for your overall well-being. Remember to check with your doctor before starting any exercise program.

- **Drink lots of water.** Water can help get your digestion moving if you're constipated and helps you rehydrate if you're suffering from diarrhea.

- **Eat plenty of fiber.** That said, what's important is the *type* of fiber you eat. It's best to get your fiber from low-FODMAP foods, like oat bran, brown rice, quinoa, chia seeds, fruits, vegetables, and skin-on potatoes. Ask your health-care provider whether you should take a fiber supplement. Citrucel and FiberCon are tolerable on the low-FODMAP diet, but Metamucil usually isn't since it's fermentable and may cause gas.

- **Try probiotics.** Probiotics are live bacteria that help populate the gut with good bacteria. They can be found in supplements and in foods such as yogurt and kefir. Although probiotics will not cure IBS, they may reduce IBS symptoms in some people, depending on the dose and type of probiotic used. IBS can result from an imbalance of bacteria in the intestines, and probiotics can help restore that balance, so talk to your doctor or dietitian about which probiotics are right for you. Look for supplements that don't contain fructooligosaccharides (FOS) or chicory root/inulin, also called prebiotics. These are FODMAPs and can make your symptoms worse.

So, if you've completed the elimination and rechallenge phases and you're still experiencing symptoms, there might be other dietary factors to consider. Seeing a dietitian about identifying these other dietary triggers may be a good idea, especially if you're considering trialing a strict elimination-rechallenge diet. (That said, following a low-FODMAP diet can still be helpful even if you do find that additives are triggering your symptoms.)

What to Eat on the Low-FODMAP Diet

So, what *can* you eat on the low-FODMAP diet? Plenty. As you'll see from the recipes in this book, there's so much you can do with low-FODMAP foods. Many dietitians and researchers agree that the foods listed below are generally well-tolerated. Either consult with your physician or dietitian or the Monash FODMAP app for a complete list with serving sizes.

FRUITS

Strawberries, blueberries, raspberries, bananas, oranges, and grapes are considered low-FODMAP in the appropriate serving sizes. Note that drying fruit increases the concentration of FODMAPs as the water content is reduced: for example, low-FODMAP grapes become high-FODMAP raisins.

Avoid these fruit ingredients on food labels: some fruit juices, such as pear juice and apple juice.

Am I allergic, or intolerant? Food allergies and food intolerances are not the same thing. A true *food allergy* is an immune-system reaction that may be very serious and even life-threatening. If you have a food allergy, you may break out in hives or go into anaphylactic shock when you consume the allergen. A *food intolerance*, on the other hand, is a less severe response. It's not life-threatening, and it usually affects the digestive system. For example, if you're intolerant to lactose, you may experience gas, pain, or similar symptoms if you consume lactose containing dairy products.

VEGETABLES

Examples of low-FODMAP vegetables are carrots, certain lettuces and greens, tomatoes, zucchini, potatoes, bell peppers, and the green parts of scallions. Be aware of the serving sizes for vegetables. The cruciferous vegetables (cabbage, broccoli, and Brussels sprouts) are known for causing gas, but they're considered tolerable in small amounts. Don't eat more than the recommended serving during the elimination phase of the diet.

Avoid these vegetable ingredients on food labels: onion powder, dehydrated onion, garlic powder, and dehydrated garlic.

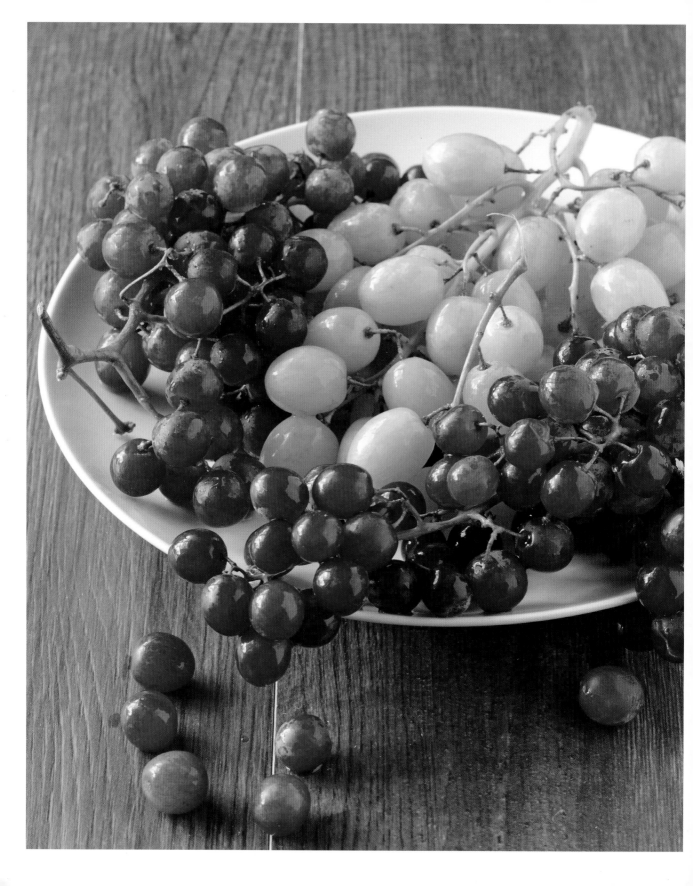

GRAINS AND CEREALS

Rice, quinoa, and cornmeal are excellent low-FODMAP grain choices. Researchers at Monash have tested the FODMAP content of starches such as tapioca, corn, and potato—all of which are generally considered well tolerated. Oats and amaranth are an exception: They have moderate levels of FODMAPs, so be mindful of the serving sizes for these grains.

If the following are major ingredients in grain-based products, you may need to limit your intake or avoid consumption during the strict elimination phase of the diet: wheat, Kamut, spelt, and sprouted wheat. This said, food processing affects FODMAP content and Monash has found some spelt sourdough breads to be low FODMAP, if they're made using a long fermentation period. Also look out for chicory root/inulin, high-fructose corn syrup, honey, agave, and molasses.

MEATS

Since animal proteins such as beef, chicken, and fish consist mainly of protein and contain very few carbohydrates, they're very low in FODMAPs. But be wary of processed meats such as sausage and deli meat. Always check the list of ingredients before you buy.

Avoid these ingredients on food labels of meat-based products: garlic and onion.

LEGUMES AND SOY

Most legumes are not low-FODMAP because of GOS, but canned lentils are more tolerable because the FODMAPs leach out into the liquid, which is then drained off before use.

Whether or not soy products are low-FODMAP is a complicated topic. Soy milk is considered low-FODMAP if it is made from soy protein rather than the whole soybean. Unfortunately, most soy milk in the United States is made from whole soybeans, so it is *not* low-FODMAP. As for tofu, if it comes in a block, it's probably low-FODMAP. Tofu is made by curdling soy milk with a coagulant; then, it's cut into blocks and drained. Most of the FODMAPs are contained in the liquid that's drained off, making block tofu generally tolerable. However, tofu also comes in a silken variety, from which the liquid is not drained. While silken tofu hasn't yet been tested, it's probably best to avoid it during the elimination phase of the diet. But the good news is that tempeh (made from fermented soybeans) and soy sauce are low-FODMAP.

Avoid these ingredients on food labels of soy-based products: soybeans, soy milk, peas, and beans that aren't tolerated.

DAIRY AND NONDAIRY SUBSTITUTES

If you are lactose-intolerant, lactose-free milk is an excellent low-FODMAP choice, and it's widely available in supermarkets. While there are a growing number of nondairy milks on the market today, you should talk to your dietitian about choosing one that's right for you.

As for cheese, remember that not all cheese is laden with lactose. The fact is, most hard cheeses, such as Cheddar and Swiss, contain very little lactose. Check the nutrition label: If the amount of total carbohydrates listed is zero, then the cheese contains little to no lactose. Softer cheeses, like ricotta and cottage cheese, do have more lactose, so limit your consumption of these during the elimination phase.

Nondairy yogurts are easier to find these days, but pay attention to their ingredients: they often contain chicory root or inulin. Also, watch out for yogurts that are sweetened with honey, agave, and fruit juices such as pear and apple.

Avoid these ingredients on dairy food labels: chicory root, inulin, honey, agave, high fructose corn syrup, and fruit juices.

FATS AND OILS

Although butter is a dairy product, it is considered low-FODMAP because it contains very little lactose. All other oils are considered low-FODMAP because they are carbohydrate-free. Nonetheless, remember that some people with IBS cannot tolerate fats in larger amounts, so keep your intake moderate.

Avoid eating excess fat: It can trigger IBS symptoms.

SWEETS AND SWEETENERS

Beware of an excess of fructose when it comes to sweeteners, for example high fructose corn syrup. Granulated sugar, also known as sucrose, consists of equal amounts of glucose (also known as dextrose or corn sugar) and fructose, so it's generally well tolerated. Molasses hasn't been tested yet, so it's best to avoid it during the elimination portion of the diet. Stevia is considered tolerable, too, but you should avoid the packets containing powdered stevia with inulin, since inulin is a FODMAP.

Chocolate lovers can rejoice: Dark chocolate is low in FODMAPs in the appropriate serving size. While there are some recipes in this book that call for chocolate chips, it is best to stick with chopped dark chocolate in the strict phase of the diet since chocolate chips have not been tested yet.

Avoid these ingredients on food labels: honey, agave nectar, high-fructose corn syrup, inulin, and sugar alcohols such as sorbitol, xylitol, and others ending in "–ol."

CONDIMENTS

Mayonnaise, Dijon mustard, and soy sauce are commonly recommended condiments on a low-FODMAP diet. Ketchup is low FODMAP in small servings (1 packet), however, larger servings may trigger IBS symptoms. (You can make your own instead: Check out my recipe for Cheeseburger and Fries Casserole with ketchup on page 142!) Only a couple types of vinegars have been tested for FODMAPs, but dietitians tend to allow most vinegars, such as red wine vinegar, on the elimination diet. In a few recipes, I do not specify a type of vinegar; in those cases, use what works best for you.

Avoid these ingredients on condiment food labels: high-fructose corn syrup, onion powder, garlic powder, inulin, and FOS.

BEVERAGES AND ALCOHOL

Since fruit consumption is fairly limited during the elimination phase, you should also avoid most fruit juices. The same goes for alcohol and caffeine. Even though some alcoholic and caffeinated beverages are low-FODMAP, such as dry wines, coffee, and green tea, alcohol and caffeine can irritate your digestive system, so try to keep consumption to a minimum.

Avoid these beverages: sweet wines, sweet alcoholic drinks such as margaritas and other drinks containing fruit juices, chicory root/inulin (found in some coffees and teas), milk products, and high-FODMAP sweeteners.

TIPS FOR VEGETARIANS AND VEGANS

IBS can affect anyone, including vegetarians and vegans. And the low-FODMAP diet can be complicated for those who avoid meat and other animal products since beans are one of the most popular forms of nonanimal protein. Most beans are forbidden during the strict phase of the low-FODMAP diet, but there are other ways for vegetarians and vegans to get the protein they need. If you're a pescetarian, fish will provide you with protein, and if you're a lacto-ovo vegetarian, you can get protein from eggs and low-lactose milk products. Vegans, however, face more of a challenge. If you're vegan, stick to small amounts of legumes, like canned lentils and chickpeas. Just be sure to limit yourself to the serving size, recommended by your dietitian or the Monash App, and spread your legume consumption over the day in order to keep your overall FODMAP load low. (And make sure the rest of your meal is strictly low-FODMAP, too.) Consider these low-FODMAP, nonanimal protein sources:

- Soft, firm, and extra-firm blocks of tofu and tempeh
- Nuts such as macadamia, peanuts, pecans, pine nuts, and walnuts
- Seeds such as pumpkin, sesame, and sunflower
- Some canned legumes, such as lentils and chickpeas (be mindful of serving sizes!)
- Quinoa and rice
- Seitan, a wheat gluten product, is a popular protein source for vegans and vegetarians—but, of course, it contains gluten. While it hasn't been tested by Monash, dietitians consider it to be low-FODMAP since gluten is a protein and not a carbohydrate. That said, if you have celiac disease or think you may have non-celiac gluten sensitivity, then it's best to avoid this product. If you're unsure, ask your doctor or dietitian whether seitan is a good choice for you.

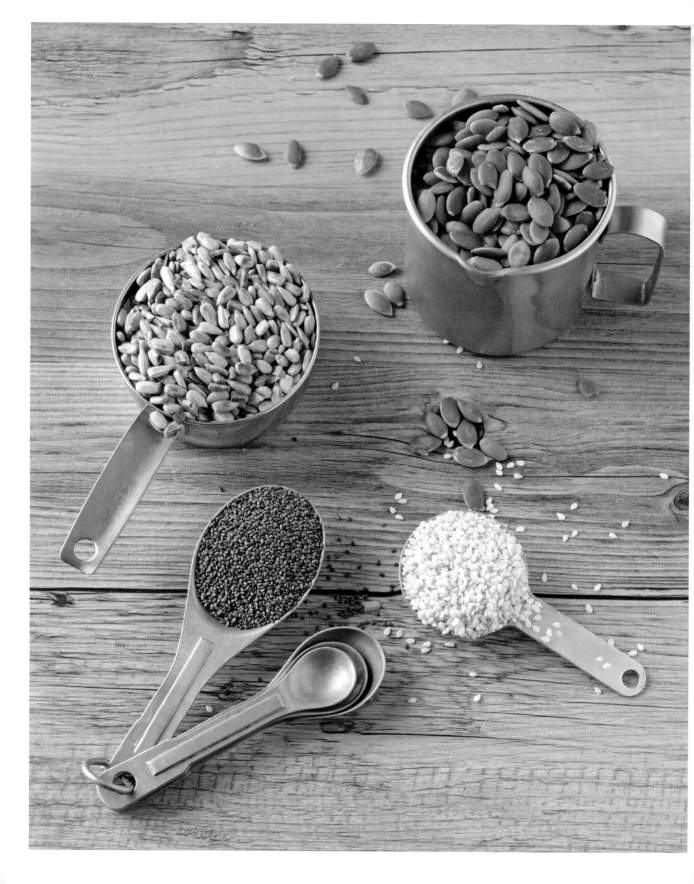

NAVIGATING THE FODMAP WORLD

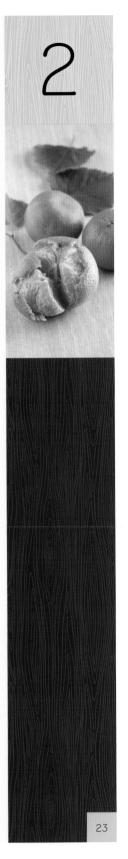

Now that you've gotten a crash course in the science behind FODMAPs and why they can aggravate IBS symptoms, you're probably wondering what this all means for your daily eating habits. This chapter will show you how to stick to low-FODMAP foods on your next trip to the grocery store; clue you in on which ingredients you should avoid on food labels; and supply you with plenty of helpful tips on eating out and choosing quick and easy low-FODMAP snacks— and lots more.

Grocery Shopping

When you're starting a low-FODMAP diet, a trip to the grocery store might feel overwhelming since it seems like *everything* has FODMAPs. It's not so! The trick is learning to read the nutrition information labels. And you'll probably find it helpful to check out your grocery store's health food section. (If your grocery store doesn't have a health food section, check out your town's food co-op or find a Whole Foods store or order nonperishable food online.) Health food or "natural food" aisles or stores are a great resource when you're looking for gluten-free foods, like gluten-free pretzels, pasta, crackers, cookies, and baking flours and mixes. And don't forget to check out the freezer section: That's where you'll find the gluten-free breads, tortillas, and pizza crusts. Remember, though, that just because a product is gluten-free doesn't mean it's low-FODMAP. Always, always be sure to read the nutrition information label.

WHICH INGREDIENTS SHOULD I AVOID?

Lots of food products do contain tricky ingredients. One of them is chicory root, otherwise known as inulin. Food companies use inulin to boost the fiber content of their products, but it can cause major tummy upset in people with digestive issues. It can turn up in anything from granola bars to packets of stevia sweeteners.

The sweeteners contained in food products can also be complicated. Sometimes manufacturers use fancy words for sweeteners to hide the fact that there is sugar in their products or to make their products seem healthier. Be on the lookout for food products sweetened with fruit juice, such as pear or apple juice. Other sweeteners to avoid are high-fructose corn syrup (regular corn syrup is fine, though),

honey, molasses, agave, and sugar alcohols (such as xylitol and sorbitol).

It can be frustrating to pick up a box of crackers that are wheat-, HFCS-, or inulin-free—only to find onion or garlic powder at the bottom of the list. Or, you might see a box of cereal that fits the bill perfectly—except for that darn honey. Don't despair, though. Eventually, you'll be able to test those foods under the guidance of your dietitian, and you may find that the amount of garlic powder or honey in them doesn't bother you. But it's best to avoid such products during the elimination phase of the diet. Also, remember that if a high-FODMAP food appears at the end of a product's ingredient list, the product could still be low-FODMAP overall. Again, check with your dietitian before you buy.

SHOP ON THE EDGE

Here's another tip to make grocery shopping easier: Stick to the outside edges of the store. This is good practice for anyone who's trying to eat healthier, but if you're avoiding FODMAPs, this is truly the key. The outside edges of the store usually feature produce, meat, cheese, and lactose-free dairy products. In the produce section, try to buy the most colorful fruits and veggies possible; more color variation means more nutrients. Invest in the fresh herbs you'll find in the produce section, too: For just a couple of dollars, you can make meals much more flavorful and exciting.

Buy unflavored, unseasoned meats, poultry, and fish in the meat case and visit the dairy aisle for hard cheeses and lactose-free milk. (Some grocery stores even have lactose-free cottage cheese and sour cream.) You can also buy lactose-free and nondairy yogurts, but beware of added high-FODMAP ingredients like inulin and fruit juices.

The grocery store's inner aisles are where all those high-FODMAP processed foods live. Of course, there are some good things to be found in those aisles, like oats, rice, rice cakes, nuts, and oils. Once you have those items, head straight to the perimeter of the store and fill up your cart. Then you can make up your own dishes from these healthy, low-FODMAP ingredients.

Food Products and Ingredients

Not all prepared food products are high-FODMAP. Here's a list of some of the great food products I like to use in my cooking. Keep an eye out for these products on your shopping trips, but be sure to keep consulting the ingredient lists on the labels because food manufacturers tend to change them frequently. Watch out for buzzwords that appear on the box, like "New and Improved!" or "New Recipe." That usually signals some ingredient changes. And consult Chapter 1 for the ingredients to look out for on package labels.

One more helpful fact: When a label lists "spices" as an ingredient, it is *not* referring to garlic and onion. According to the FDA's Code of Federal Regulations Title 21, "spices" may refer to any aromatic vegetable substance *except* for those generally regarded as "foods," such as onion, garlic, and celery. If a product contains these ingredients, they'll be listed separately.

- **Sandwich bread.** Udi's sandwich bread is found in the freezer in natural food stores. It's a low-FODMAP, gluten-free bread, and it gets great reviews. When I worked in natural foods, I noticed that it flew off the shelves! If you'd rather not make your own bread for sandwiches, croutons, and bread crumbs, it's an excellent choice.

- **Tortillas.** Corn tortillas are my go-to for wraps and tacos, and they're usually available in regular grocery stores. You can also find gluten-free tortillas by Food for Life and Rudi's in the frozen section of a natural foods store.

- **Crackers, pretzels, and chips.** Look for these low-FODMAP crackers: Sesmark Rice Thins, Crunchmaster Multi-Seed Crackers (Original), Blue Diamond Nut Thins (Almond Sea Salt and Pecan), and Mary's Gone Crackers (Original). These are my favorites, and they're wonderful with some cheddar or Swiss cheese. They're all easily found in natural foods stores. As for gluten-free pretzels, look for the Snyder's of Hanover brand. Lundberg Rice Chips (Sea Salt), plain tortilla chips, and baked potato chips are nice, crunchy low-FODMAP snack options, too, but be aware of the added fats, which may not be appropriate for some people.

- **Lactose-free and nondairy milks.** Lactaid, of course, makes lactose-free milk, in which the lactase enzyme has been added in order to break down the lactose. Coconut milk, along with lactose-free milk, has been tested by Monash University and is considered "safe" in appropriate servings. (Try to find the "light" canned variety.) Almond milk could be a possible alternative to discuss with your dietitian. Soy milk is another option, but only if it's made from the soybean extract and not the whole bean. 8th Continent is a reliable brand. (The label on the carton usually states whether or not it's made from the whole bean.) When it comes to nondairy milks in general, look out for additives, such as xanthan gum and inulin.

- **Yogurt and other dairy products.** Green Valley Organics produces organic, lactose-free, low-FODMAP yogurt and sour cream, and Lifeway plain kefir, at 99 percent lactose-free, is another great option. There are other nondairy yogurts on the market, but many are unsuitable because they have added inulin.

- **Gluten-free flours.** I'm a big fan of Bob's Red Mill. They carry just about any gluten-free flour imaginable, including brown rice flour, quinoa flour, oat flour, and potato starch. I'm sensitive to xanthan gum, so I make my own flour blends with these flours (see page 38 for my own blend recipe). But if you're not sensitive to xanthan gum, there are some great gluten-free all-purpose blends that are also low-FODMAP. (Remember, just because something is gluten-free doesn't mean that it's also low-FODMAP! Read the labels carefully.) Look for Namaste flour and baking mixes, King Arthur gluten-free flour, and Bisquick gluten-free baking mix.

- **Tomato sauce.** You wouldn't believe how difficult it can be to find plain tomato sauce without added onion or garlic. I finally came across a brand called Pomi, which is sold in aseptic containers. Their tomato sauce and diced tomatoes are 100 percent tomatoes, pure and simple. Bionaturae also makes pure tomato sauce.

- **Cereals.** Some standard low-FODMAP cereals that are found at regular grocery stores include General Mills Corn Chex (Rice Chex contains molasses, which may be high in fructose, so use caution). Visit a natural foods store for other great cereals. Erewhon makes gluten-free crisp rice cereal and gluten-free cornflakes, while Arrowhead Mills makes a lovely hot cereal called Rice and Shine. And don't forget oatmeal and quinoa flakes.

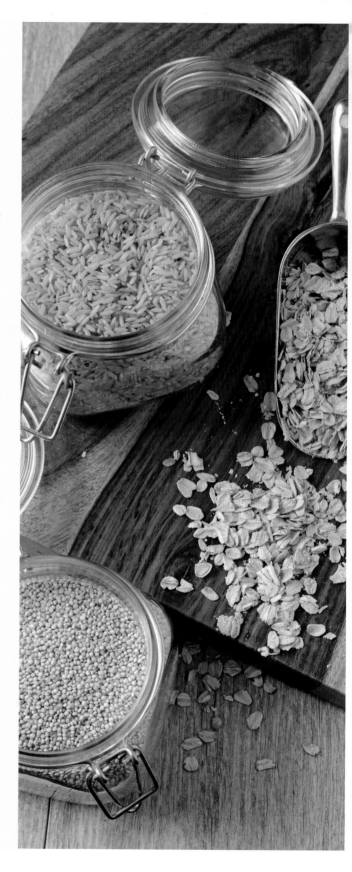

- **Pasta.** Tinkyada brown rice pastas are excellent, and Ancient Harvest also makes pasta out of quinoa and corn. Other private labels and some store brands are delving into the gluten-free pasta world, too. As always, be sure to read the label.

- **Condiments.** Butter can be used in the appropriate serving size, and Earth Balance makes a wonderful nondairy, vegan margarine that you can spread on your toast or use in baking. Hellmann's Real Mayonnaise is low-FODMAP, but I actually prefer Vegenaise, a vegan mayo alternative, since I'm sensitive to eggs. Organic fruit spreads, such as strawberry or blueberry jam, are best because they're sweetened with sugar, not HFCS. Other condiments to keep on hand include San-J gluten-free tamari and Dijon mustard. And I can't say it often enough: Don't forget to check the ingredients lists!

Eating Out on the Low-FODMAP Diet

Now you know how to navigate the grocery store—but what about eating out? Don't worry: Sticking to a low-FODMAP diet when you're dining out is totally doable. Here are some tips for making eating at restaurants easier.

- **Check out the menu online.** Scope out the menu and decide what to order ahead of time. Consider calling the restaurant in advance to ask whether they accommodate special diets. With the rise in celiac and food intolerance diagnoses, lots of restaurants are becoming more flexible, so it's likely that you'll be pleasantly surprised.

- **Contact your local celiac support group.** When I lived in St. Cloud, Minnesota, the local celiac support group had created a list of restaurants that offered gluten-free options or that were willing to work with you to create a meal you could eat. You may not be celiac, but these groups can still be excellent resources.

- **Don't be afraid to talk to your server or to the chef.** Most restaurant professionals are used to accommodating patrons with allergies and food sensitivities.

- **Stick with basic, simple dishes.** Think grilled, steamed, or broiled salmon, chicken, or steak. Baked potatoes, undressed salads, and steamed veggies are also good choices. Ask your server to hold the garlic or onion and stick to salt and pepper for seasonings.

- **Bring your own salad dressing.** I have a set of little plastic containers that are the perfect size for holding my own dressings. Invest in a set of your own—or, simply ask for a plain oil and vinegar dressing on your salad. (You could even bring your own vegan margarine for a baked potato, if you like.)

- **Bring your own bread**—or your own hamburger bun.

- **Suggest having a potluck dinner** instead of going out and then bring a low-FODMAP dish to share. Who knows—you might introduce a friend or family member to a new way of eating in the process!

Low-FODMAP Snack Ideas

I don't know about you, but I need to eat snacks throughout the day to boost my energy levels—and to stop my stomach from growling! Here are some easy snack ideas that'll help you keep hunger at bay.

- **Rice cakes.** Top a plain rice cake with peanut butter and sliced fresh strawberries.

- **Roll-ups.** Whip up a quick, filling snack by rolling up a gluten-free tortilla with sliced turkey, Swiss cheese, and mayo or with peanut butter and organic raspberry jam.

- **Nuts and seeds.** This one couldn't be easier: Simply grab a handful of some low-FODMAP nuts or seeds, such as walnuts, pecans, or pumpkin seeds.

- **Fruits and veggies.** Nosh on a suitable serving size of low-FODMAP fruit, like mandarins, strawberries, ripe banana, or cantaloupe, or crunch on some carrot sticks.

- **Cheese and crackers.** This is one of my all-time favorite snacks! Pair gluten-free rice crackers or gluten-free pretzels with cheddar cheese slices.

- **Granola Bars (page 174), Power Poppers (page 183), Graham-Style Crackers (page 182), or Granola (pages 46 and 48).** These slightly sweet snacks are so satisfying, and the best part is, you won't end up with a sugar crash later in the day. Plus, they're portable, so they're easy to take with you to work or school.

- **Muffins or banana bread** (page 62) make fabulous morning snacks, especially with a cup of coffee.

- **Smoothies.** Just toss a few healthy ingredients into a blender, and you're ready to go. Check out the Banana Smoothie, Three Ways on page 173.

Meal Planning

Planning and organizing come naturally to me. Believe it or not, I love putting together grocery lists and menu plans! And I've come up with a routine that makes eating a varied, flavorful, low-FODMAP diet simple, low-stress, and enjoyable.

My meal planning starts on Saturday. In the morning, I make up my menu for the following week by jotting down my ideas on a sheet of paper. Then I turn the paper over and make a grocery list based on my ideas. Dinners are usually my main focus; then, I make sure that we're well stocked on the basics, so that my husband and I can make our usual breakfasts and lunches. I also like to keep an eye on what's on sale at the grocery store and on the types of produce that are in season.

Weekends are when I make more complicated meals, since I have plenty of time. I also like to make my stocks, broths, and soups on weekends: I freeze stocks and broth in different-sized containers, depending upon the amounts called for in the recipes I plan on preparing. And I like to freeze soups in single-serving containers so that I can thaw and heat them easily for weekday lunches.

Lazy Sundays are also a great time to make weekday breakfasts in advance, like egg cups, frittatas, pancakes, or waffles. It's simple to freeze pancakes or waffles: Just lay them in a single layer on a baking sheet and place in the freezer. When the pancakes or waffles are frozen, transfer them into a plastic freezer bag and store in the freezer. Then pop them in the microwave whenever a craving strikes.

There are plenty of delicious lunch options in my meal plans, too, like sandwiches made with gluten-free bread and salads. Feel free to add extra protein to any of my salads; grilled chicken or salmon will make them even better!

	BREAKFAST	LUNCH	DINNER
SUNDAY	Banana Bread Brown Rice Porridge (page 58)	Greek Quinoa Salad (page 85)	Red Wine Oven Pot Roast with Thyme Gravy (page 140)
MONDAY	Zucchini Quinoa Egg Muffins (page 60)	Leftover pot roast sandwich with gluten-free bread	Baked Tilapia with Greek Blistered-Tomato Pasta (page 102)
TUESDAY	Gluten-free cornflakes with sliced bananas and lactose-free milk	Chicken Soup (page 113)	Maple-Marinated Salmon with Sesame Spinach Rice (page 151)
WEDNESDAY	Peanut Butter Overnight Quinoa and Oats (page 50)	Greek Quinoa Salad (page 85)	Hearty Meatloaf (page 146) with Parmesan Garlic Smashed Potatoes (page 88) and green beans
THURSDAY	Scrambled eggs or Tofu Scrambled Rancheros (page 61) and gluten-free toast	Caesar Salad (page 83) with grilled chicken breast	Sautéed Chicken with Dijon Sauce (page 127) with Rosemary Roasted Red Potatoes (page 89) and Balsamic and Blue Spinach Salad (page 81)
FRIDAY	Very Berry Granola (page 49) with lactose-free milk	Chicken Salad with Pecans and Grapes (page 86) with gluten-free crackers	Classic Supreme Pizza (page 165)
SATURDAY	Pancakes (pages 53 and 54)	Oven-Fried Chicken Fingers with Maple Mustard Dipping Sauce (page 128)	Shrimp Pasta with Lemon and Kale (page 157)

Following is a couple weeks' worth of sample menus. These are just examples of the meal plans you can create for yourself and your family using the recipes in this book, so don't feel that you have to follow them to the letter!

I'm a big fan of leftovers, so most of these recipes are designed to feed four people—even though I'm usually just cooking for my husband and myself. That means that I only have to cook half as many dinners during the week, which definitely makes life easier. Or, if you have a bigger family, you can easily double the recipe and plan on eating the leftovers the following evening or for lunch. When I was a kid, I hated leftovers, but now, I can't imagine life without them!

SAMPLE MENU: WEEK 2

	BREAKFAST	LUNCH	DINNER
SUNDAY	Potato Frittata (page 59)	Turkey and Swiss sandwich on gluten-free bread with carrot sticks	Lemon and Thyme Roasted Chicken (page 126) with Parmesan Garlic Smashed Potatoes (page 88) and green beans
MONDAY	Quinoa flakes hot cereal with cinnamon and blueberries	Sautéed Zucchini Pasta (page 105) with sautéed chicken	Beef Tacos (page 148) and Cilantro Lime Rice (page 100)
TUESDAY	Scrambled eggs or Tofu Scrambled Rancheros (page 61) and gluten-free toast	Raspberry Walnut Salad (page 82) with grilled salmon	Salmon Chowder (page 118) with Maple Cinnamon Corn Bread (page 77)
WEDNESDAY	Peanut Butter Overnight Quinoa and Oats (page 50)	Chicken Soup (page 113)	Creamy Pesto Tuna Pasta (page 153) with Caesar Salad (page 83)
THURSDAY	Zucchini and Quinoa Egg Muffins (page 60)	Turkey Keema with Veggies (page 139) over rice	Grilled Marinated Pork Chops (page 159) and Baked Brown Rice with Parmesan and Herbs (page 97)
FRIDAY	Pumpkin Pecan Granola (page 46) with lactose-free milk	Spinach Quinoa Tabbouleh (page 96)	Chicken Pesto Pizza (page 165)
SATURDAY	Pumpkin Spice Waffles (page 57) and bacon	Oven-Fried Chicken Fingers with Maple Mustard Dipping Sauce (page 128)	Crispy Baked Cod (page 149) with Citrus Fennel Carrot Slaw (page 80)

Adding Flavor to Low-FODMAP Food

Low-FODMAP food doesn't have to be bland—far from it! Over the past couple of years, I've figured out how to add plenty of flavor to my dishes, and these days, I don't miss onion or garlic at all. Boost flavor in your low-FODMAP meals by using the following:

- **Salt and pepper.** I know, it seems so basic, but using salt and pepper is absolutely essential. Often, when a dish tastes bland, it's not because it's lacking garlic or onion, but because it's lacking salt. Luckily, salt is not a FODMAP. I'm not suggesting that you eat a high-sodium diet, but keep in mind that Americans get most of their sodium from processed foods. And if you're reducing your intake of processed foods (as you probably will be if you're on a low-FODMAP diet), then adding more salt to your cooking isn't terribly worrisome. However, salt shouldn't be used with abandon, especially if your doctor has recommended a lower sodium intake. Follow my lead and use just enough salt to give the dish flavor. Balance is the key.

- **Chives and scallions.** If you love the flavor of onions, chives and scallions can supply your fix. Just be sure to use the green parts only. For the most pungent flavor, use them raw and sprinkle them over a dish just before serving.

- **Garlic oil.** Garlic is high in fructans, but guess what? Fructans aren't soluble in oil. That means it's fine to simmer garlic in oil to infuse the oil with its wonderful flavor. But beware: The fructans in garlic and onion *are* soluble in water, which means the fructans can leach out into the water they're cooking in. That's why you should never use garlic or onion in broths or soups; only use it to flavor oil! Make your own garlic oil at home and consume it right after you make it since harmful bacteria can flourish in the leftover oil.

- **Herbs and spices.** Lots of herbs and spices are low-FODMAP, and they're a great way to pep up soups and slow cooker meals. Try adding some freshly chopped parsley or cilantro to dishes before serving and use spices like cinnamon in savory dishes, such as Turkey Keema with Veggies (see page 139).

- **Lemons, limes, and citrus zest.** Freshly squeezed lemon and lime juices add a palate-lifting burst of flavor to lots of dishes—and for an even more intense citrus hit, you can add freshly grated citrus zest, too. I really love my Microplane zester: I even use it to add orange flavor to cookies or my Cranberry Orange Scones (see page 66).

- **Broths and stocks.** Chicken, beef, and vegetable broths aren't just for soups: They're great flavor enhancers, especially in tasty sauces. I used to think making broth and stock was really complicated, but it turns out it's practically foolproof. Just throw some chicken bones and veggies in a pot of water and simmer away. The more you make it, the easier it gets. Beef stock does require an extra step—the bones have to be roasted first—but it's so worth it. Freeze the broth in different-sized containers so it's recipe-ready when you need it. (For very small amounts, try freezing the broth in an ice cube tray or muffin pan.)

- **Umami ingredients.** The word *umami* describes a sort of savory meatiness, and adding a dash of umami to a dish enhances the flavors of the ingredients. Beef broth is both low-FODMAP and umami and so is gluten-free soy sauce, tamari, anchovies, olives, and Parmesan cheese. Add them to marinades, sauces, salads—or just about any dish you can think of.

- **Dry wines.** Dry wines are actually low-FODMAP—in moderation, of course. In the kitchen, they can be used in sauces, stews, and slow cooker meals. Or, use a splash of wine to deglaze the pan after you've browned meat, as part of creating a delicious sauce.

- **Toasted grains and nuts.** I often skip this step if I'm in a hurry, but I always regret it! Toasting rice and quinoa before cooking it really brings out the grains' beautiful nutty flavor. The same goes for nuts and seeds, like walnuts, pine nuts, or sunflower seeds. Toss them in a dry skillet over medium heat before sprinkling them on salads.

Great Gluten-Free Baking

Gluten-free baking can be a little tricky, but with practice, you can definitely master it. I've been experimenting with gluten-free flours for several years now. I've had some successes (and plenty of failures!), and in the process, I've I accumulated some tips for making gluten-free baking easier.

First, none of my recipes call for xanthan gum, which is often used to help give gluten-free baked goods more structure, resulting in better rising and less crumbling. That's because I developed a sensitivity to xanthan gum, which, as I discovered, isn't that uncommon. And I figured that, since most of my readers already have delicate bellies, they certainly don't need yet another sensitivity added to the mix. So, all my recipes have been designed and tested to work without xanthan gum.

You'll also want to pay attention to the type of flour you use. I find that a mixture of flours works consistently—usually a combination of starch and protein flours. Starch flours have very little protein or fiber and are very white and powdery. These include potato starch, cornstarch, and tapioca flour. Potato starch and cornstarch are good for making things that are crisp and crunchy, like cookies and crackers. Tapioca flour helps keep cakes and breads moist and spongy. Ultimately, using a blend of starch flours helps make a good all-purpose flour.

Protein flours, of course, have protein in them. They also contain fiber, especially the whole-grain kinds, and they're made by grinding up whole grains, such as rice, oats, and quinoa. A combination of protein and starch flours is usually best in most recipes: I find that a ratio of 2 parts protein flour to 1 part starch flour works well.

The way in which gluten-free flours are measured is very important, too. Most gluten-free baking purists swear that weighing each and every type of flour is the only way to go. But I grew up using measuring cups, and while I do own a scale, I still find the measuring cups easier to use. Nonetheless, it's still really important to measure the flour correctly. Start by scooping the flour *into* the measuring cup (scooping the flour *with* the measuring cup itself tends to compact the flour, which means you're adding too much flour to your recipe). Use a spoon or scoop to lightly fill the measuring cup until it's overflowing. Then level it off using the back of a knife.

When I'm making breads, I like to bake smaller loaves. The typical bread pan is usually 5 x 9 inches (13 x 23 cm), but I use a 4 x 8-inch (10 x 20 cm) pan for all of my breads since smaller loaves bake more evenly. Plus, since they're smaller, the loaf is less likely to collapse. These pans are fairly easy to find, too: I bought mine at the local grocery store.

Finally, mixing the batter or dough really well is very important. When you bake with wheat, recipes often caution you against overmixing since this produces too much gluten and turns out tough, chewy baked goods. But when you're using gluten-free

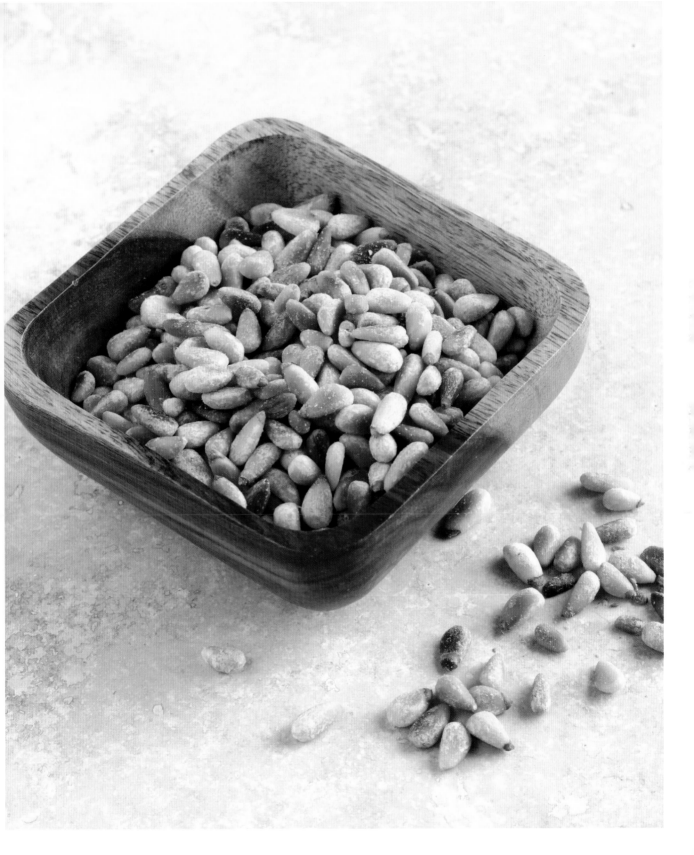

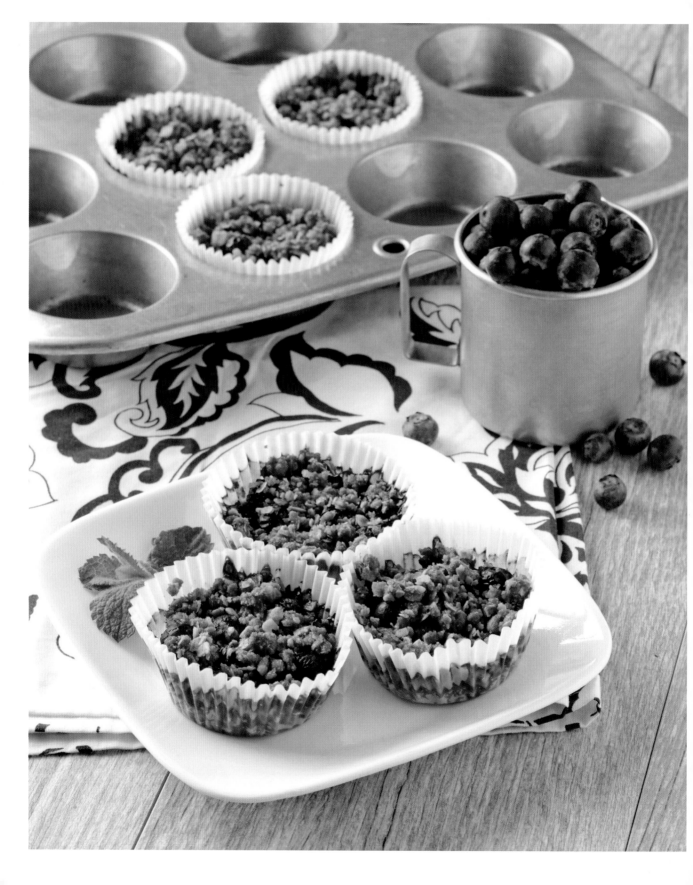

flours, you don't have to worry about producing too much gluten. In fact, it's best to mix all of the ingredients as thoroughly as possible since incorporating more air into the dough results in a lighter loaf of bread.

Because of the nature of gluten-free baked goods, and because I don't use any gums in my recipes, they do tend to dry out fairly rapidly. That's why I usually freeze my bread, muffins, and scones within a day or two of baking. Then I just take what I need out of the freezer and thaw it. If your baked goods do dry out, often you can "revive" or soften them by microwaving them for a few seconds.

Adapting Your Own Recipes to a Low-FODMAP Diet

Here's some good news: Lots of your favorite recipes can be made low-FODMAP, and you can adapt them yourself! First of all, it's important to adapt the right recipes. It really helps if the recipe's main ingredient is already low-FODMAP. For example, a chicken soup recipe is a lot easier to adapt than a French onion soup recipe! Chicken is low-FODMAP, but onions are decidedly not, and the recipe wouldn't make sense without them. So, try to stick to recipes that are based around a low-FODMAP food.

Second, be aware of possible substitutions. For example, you can use gluten-free flour blend in place of wheat flour in sauces and baked goods. Or, you can use maple syrup instead of honey; substitute lactose-free or nondairy milk for regular milk; and use pine nuts in place of cashews. Sauté meat in homemade garlic oil instead of adding minced garlic to the mix. Use the green parts of scallions instead of regular onions. Try gluten-free noodles in pasta recipes. Cut gluten-free, low-FODMAP bread into cubes and dry them in the oven to make croutons, stuffing, and bread crumbs. Or, look for alternatives to bread crumbs, like crushed gluten-free crackers or cereal. Make homemade cream sauces using low-FODMAP ingredients instead of using canned, condensed cream soups in casseroles. (If this sounds like a lot to remember, don't worry: There are plenty of examples of these substitutions in the recipes that follow.)

Third, be mindful of the overall FODMAP content of a recipe. Some foods are considered low-FODMAP, but only in the recommended serving size. For instance, the suggested serving size for broccoli is half a cup (36 g), but larger servings contain GOS (galactans). So, it might not be a good idea to combine broccoli with another food that contains GOS, such as lentils, since a couple of small servings of two different foods eaten at the same time can add up to a large overall serving of GOS. The recipes in this book are as well balanced in this way as possible, and I hope they inspire you to create new low-FODMAP recipes and to adapt your tried-and-true favorites.

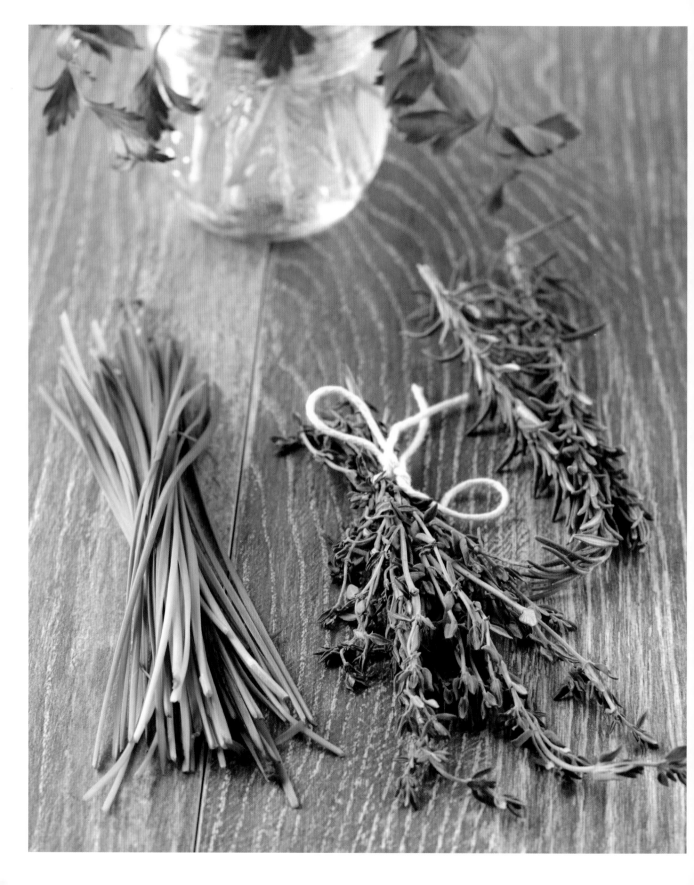

THE BASICS

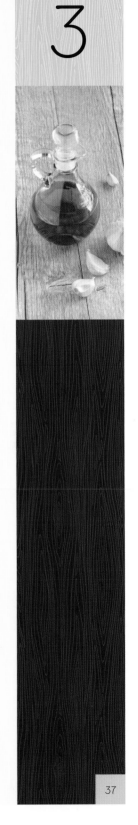

3

Before you start making these low-FODMAP recipes, you'll want to have a few homemade basics on hand. One of the most essential staple ingredients is my Basic Flour Blend on page 38. It's a wheat- and gluten-free flour mixture that's also free of gums and additives, and it pops up in dozens of recipes in this book, either as a thickener (it's great for making soups and stews thick and creamy) or as a base for low-FODMAP baked goods, like breads, muffins, and cookies. You'll also find that there are plenty of ways to add flavor to low-FODMAP dishes, and that's where my Homemade Garlic Oil (page 42) and Herb Seasonings (page 40) come in. Garlic isn't low-FODMAP, but since its fructans won't leach into the hot oil, it's safe to enjoy in lots of low-FODMAP savory dishes. (Just be sure to store your Homemade Garlic Oil according to the tips on page 42.) And you'll want to whip up a batch of my Spinach Basil Pesto (page 41), too. You can pair it with pasta, of course, but it's also fabulous as a pizza topping or stirred into vegetables. In fact, you'll want to add it to just about everything!

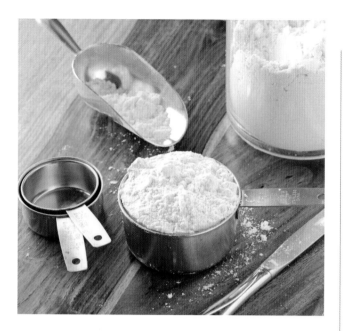

BASIC FLOUR BLEND

YIELD: ABOUT 3½ CUPS (568 G)

This versatile flour blend is great in pancakes, cookies, and muffins, and it works as a sauce and gravy thickener, too. Since I omit gums, such as xanthan and guar, in my recipes, it's good to know that replacing some of the flour blend with more tapioca flour adds lift and elasticity to breads—and the extra tapioca flour also keeps biscuits and scones from being too crumbly. Finally, brown rice flour provides a hefty dose of fiber.

2½ CUPS (400 G) BROWN RICE FLOUR

½ CUP (96 G) POTATO STARCH

⅓ CUP (40 G) TAPIOCA FLOUR

¼ CUP (32 G) CORNSTARCH

Measure each ingredient by lightly spooning the flour into the measuring cup until overflowing and then use the back of a knife to level off the flour. (Use this same method when you're measuring this flour blend for recipes.) Blend the ingredients thoroughly with a spoon and store in an airtight container in the refrigerator for up to several months.

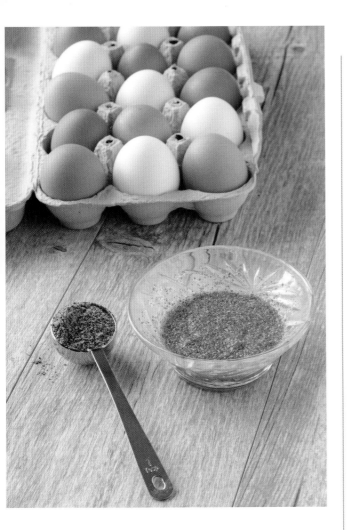

CHIA EGG REPLACER

YIELD: MAKES 1 CHIA EGG, THE EQUIVALENT OF 1 LARGE EGG

When they're soaked in water, chia seeds form a gelatinous mixture that's very similar in texture to eggs. So, once I realized that I couldn't tolerate eggs, I started using this egg replacer, which works really well in as a binding agent in my Hearty Meatloaf (page 146) and in meatballs (see Italian Wedding Soup on page 117 and Swedish Chicken Meatballs on page 136). It's also great for baking—just keep in mind that the Chia Egg Replacer only works in recipes that call for one egg or two at the most.

Use a clean coffee grinder to grind the chia seeds. Using ground seeds makes the mixture form a gel more quickly and helps the seeds become thoroughly incorporated into the other ingredients. Chia seeds can also be used to replace xanthan gum in some of my recipes, like the Gingerbread Biscotti on page 171.

1 TABLESPOON (13 G) FINELY GROUND CHIA SEEDS

¼ CUP (60 ML) WARM WATER

In a small bowl, whisk together the ground chia seed and water. Let the mixture sit until it forms a gel-like consistency, about 5 minutes. Use in your recipes in place of an egg.

HERB SEASONINGS

YIELD: ABOUT ¼ CUP (12 G) EACH

Herbs are a wonderful way to add flavor to your cooking. I rely on dried herbs, which are inexpensive and convenient, but if you prefer to use fresh herbs, go right ahead! These blends complement a number of the dishes in this book, like the Zucchini Quinoa Egg Muffins on page 60, and the Walnut-Crusted Chicken Parmesan on page 130, but feel free to alter them to suit your preferences, if you like. And they couldn't be easier to make: Simply combine the herbs and then store the mixture in your pantry in an airtight container for maximum freshness. Both of these blends are designed to fit into the typical spice jars found at kitchen supply stores.

Italian Herb Seasoning

1 TABLESPOON (3 G) DRIED OREGANO

1 TABLESPOON (3 G) DRIED THYME

2 TEASPOONS CRUSHED DRIED ROSEMARY

2 TEASPOONS DRIED BASIL

1 TEASPOON DRIED MARJORAM

1 TEASPOON DRIED RUBBED SAGE

Poultry Herb Seasoning

2 TABLESPOONS (3 G) DRIED PARSLEY

1 TABLESPOON (2 G) DRIED RUBBED SAGE

1½ TEASPOONS CRUSHED DRIED ROSEMARY

1½ TEASPOONS DRIED MARJORAM

For each herb blend, just mix the herbs until well combined and then store in an airtight container.

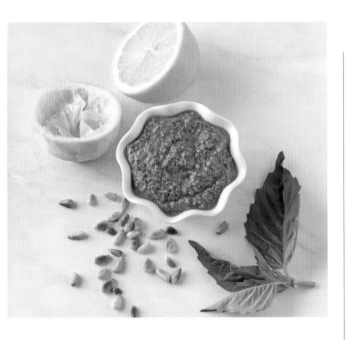

SPINACH BASIL PESTO

YIELD: ABOUT 1 CUP (235 ML)

This pesto is in the Basics chapter because it's so darn versatile. And it's not just for tossing with pasta. Sure, you can use it to create a creamy pasta sauce, as in Creamy Pesto Tuna Pasta on page 153—but you can also use it on pizza (check out the Chicken Pesto Pizza on page 165) or add it to egg dishes (try the Pesto Potato Frittata on page 59). My recipe uses garlic oil in place of the traditional garlic cloves, and it's absolutely packed with flavor.

½ CUP (120 ML) EXTRA-VIRGIN OLIVE OIL

4 CLOVES OF GARLIC, PEELED AND SMASHED, BUT KEPT WHOLE

1½ CUPS (45 G) BABY SPINACH LEAVES

¾ CUP (18 G) FRESH BASIL LEAVES

½ CUP (70 G) PINE NUTS, TOASTED OR ¼ CUP (36 G) SUNFLOWER SEEDS, TOASTED

½ CUP (50 G) GRATED PARMESAN CHEESE (OPTIONAL)

½ TEASPOON KOSHER SALT

½ TEASPOON FRESHLY GROUND BLACK PEPPER

½ TEASPOON LEMON ZEST

1 TABLESPOON (15 ML) FRESH LEMON JUICE

Since pesto contains garlic oil, you should store and use it in the same way you'd use the Homemade Garlic Oil on page 42 in order to avoid harmful bacteria growth.

Heat the olive oil in a skillet over medium heat. Add the garlic and sauté until browned. Remove the garlic and discard. Let the oil cool to room temperature.

To a food processor, add the spinach, basil, pine nuts, Parmesan cheese (if using), kosher salt, black pepper, lemon zest, and lemon juice. Add 2 tablespoons (28 ml) of the cooled garlic oil. Process until almost smooth. With the processor running, slowly pour in the rest of the garlic oil. Scrape down the sides of the processor bowl if necessary and process again.

Use as desired immediately or freeze. To freeze, pour the pesto evenly into an ice cube tray. Wrap the tray in plastic wrap and freeze. Once frozen, remove the cubes from the tray and store in a heavy-duty plastic freezer bag. Use as needed.

HOMEMADE GARLIC OIL

YIELD: VARIES

I love garlic, so this homemade infused oil is one of my low-FODMAP kitchen staples. Garlic is high in fructans, but they aren't oil-soluble, so sautéing garlic in oil releases its pungent flavor, but, luckily, not the fructans. Still, it's best to consult your doctor or dietitian first to decide whether garlic oil is a good option for you. Use a proportion of 1 clove of garlic per 1 to 2 tablespoons (15 to 28 ml) of oil for this recipe, scaling up as necessary. Any oil will work, but I like olive oil the best.

Because of the risk of bacteria growth, you should consume your Homemade Garlic Oil within a day or two, just to be on the safe side. Store it in the refrigerator if you're not going to use it immediately and consume it within 2 to 4 days. Alternatively, you can freeze it for up to 3 months. The best way to do this is to freeze the oil in a clean ice cube tray: That way, you can add the individual portions of oil directly to your recipes without having to let it thaw.

WHOLE CLOVES OF GARLIC

OIL OF YOUR CHOICE, SUCH AS OLIVE, CANOLA, OR WALNUT

Place the garlic on a cutting board and lay the flat side of chef's knife down on top of the cloves. Whack the knife with the heel of your hand, smashing the cloves of garlic. Not only does this peel the garlic, but it also smashes it, making it easier to release the garlic flavors when sautéing in oil.

Heat the oil in a skillet or saucepan over medium heat. Add the peeled garlic and sauté until it starts to brown, about 1½ to 2 minutes. Remove the garlic from the oil and discard. Let the oil cool and then use it in your favorite recipes. Consume the oil immediately or refrigerate it for up to 2 days.

Using Homemade Garlic Oil Safely
Never store garlic oil at room temperature. Always keep it in the refrigerator and discard any unused oil after a few days. The best, and safest, way to use frozen garlic oil is to add individual portions of the frozen oil directly to your recipe without defrosting it first.

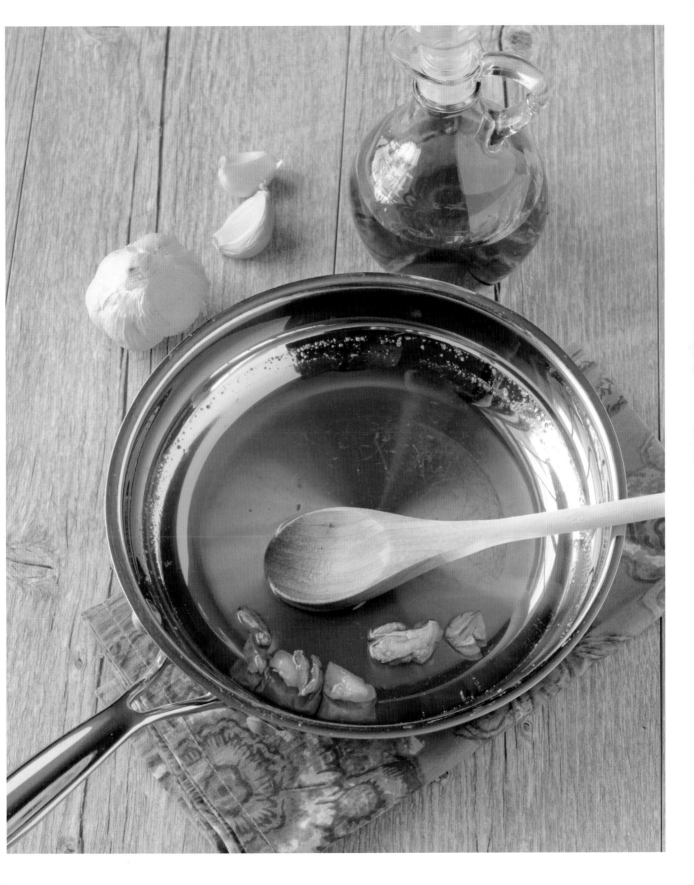

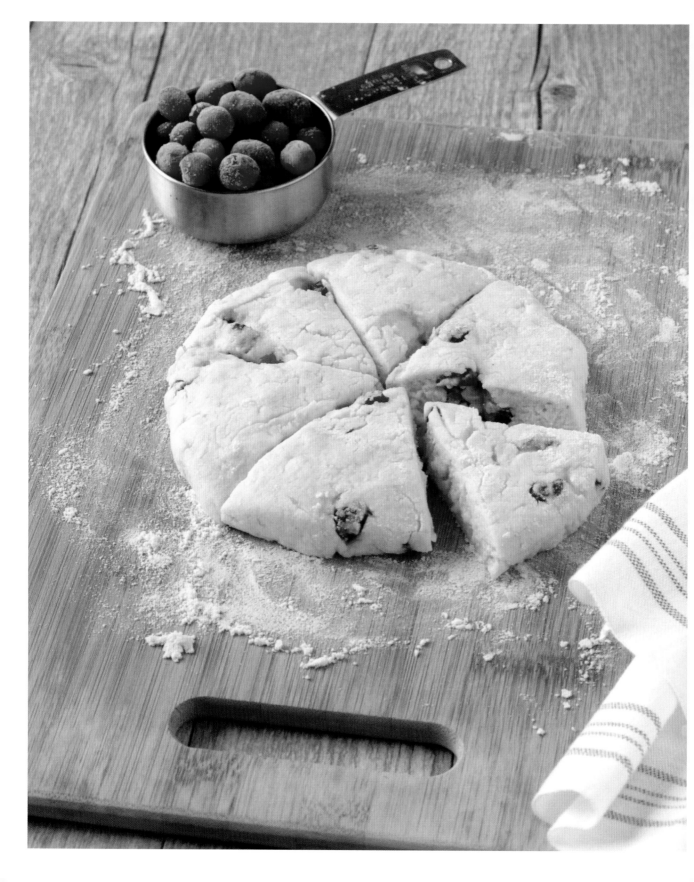

BREAKFAST, BREADS, AND MUFFINS

4

I'm a die-hard breakfast lover, and I completely agree with the famous phrase that calls it the most important meal of the day. If you can't live without your morning meal, either, I've got you covered. This chapter features recipes for porridge, granola, and cereals, which make for easy breakfasts during the workweek—plus inventive ways to whip up low-FODMAP pancakes, waffles, and egg dishes on the weekends.

If you're vegan, you'll be glad to hear that many, if not most, of my recipes are vegan-friendly. The Tofu Scramble Rancheros on page 61 is naturally vegan, and other recipes can easily be made dairy- and egg-free, too, like the Fluffy Blueberry Pancakes on page 54. If you're looking for something lighter to enjoy with your morning coffee or tea, you'll want to try my recipes for breads, muffins, and scones. (The Banana Bread on page 62 and the quinoa-based Morning Glory Muffins on page 69 are two of my favorites!) And, for a holiday treat, look no further than the gluten-free Cranberry Orange Scones on page 66.

PUMPKIN PECAN GRANOLA

YIELD: 9 SERVINGS, ⅔ CUP (67 G) EACH

This granola is the perfect start to a crisp fall morning. Try not to overindulge, though: Since oats contain a moderate amount of FODMAPs, be sure to stick to the suggested serving size. Eat it by the handful or douse it with lactose-free milk and enjoy it as a breakfast cereal.

2 CUPS (160 G) QUICK-COOKING OATS (GLUTEN-FREE, IF NECESSARY)

2 CUPS (68 G) GLUTEN-FREE CRISPY RICE CEREAL (SUCH AS EREWHON—CHECK PRODUCT INGREDIENTS FOR FODMAPS)

1 CUP (102 G) QUINOA FLAKES

½ CUP (55 G) COARSELY CHOPPED PECANS

½ CUP (80 G) RAW PEPITAS (HULLED PUMPKIN SEEDS)

1 TEASPOON GROUND CINNAMON

½ TEASPOON GROUND GINGER

¼ TEASPOON GROUND NUTMEG

⅛ TEASPOON GROUND CLOVES

¼ TEASPOON SALT

½ CUP (120 ML) PURE MAPLE SYRUP

¼ CUP (60 ML) CANOLA OIL OR OTHER NEUTRAL OIL

¼ CUP (60 ML) WATER

Preheat the oven to 350°F (180°C, or gas mark 4). Line a rimmed baking sheet with parchment paper. In a large bowl, combine the oats, rice cereal, quinoa flakes, pecans, pepitas, cinnamon, ginger, nutmeg, ground cloves, and salt. In a small bowl, whisk together the maple syrup, canola oil, and water. Pour over the oat mixture and stir until all the oats, nuts, and seeds are coated.

Spread the mixture evenly on the prepared baking sheet. Bake for 30 minutes, stirring every 10 minutes, until lightly toasted. Let cool completely. Store in an airtight container for several weeks.

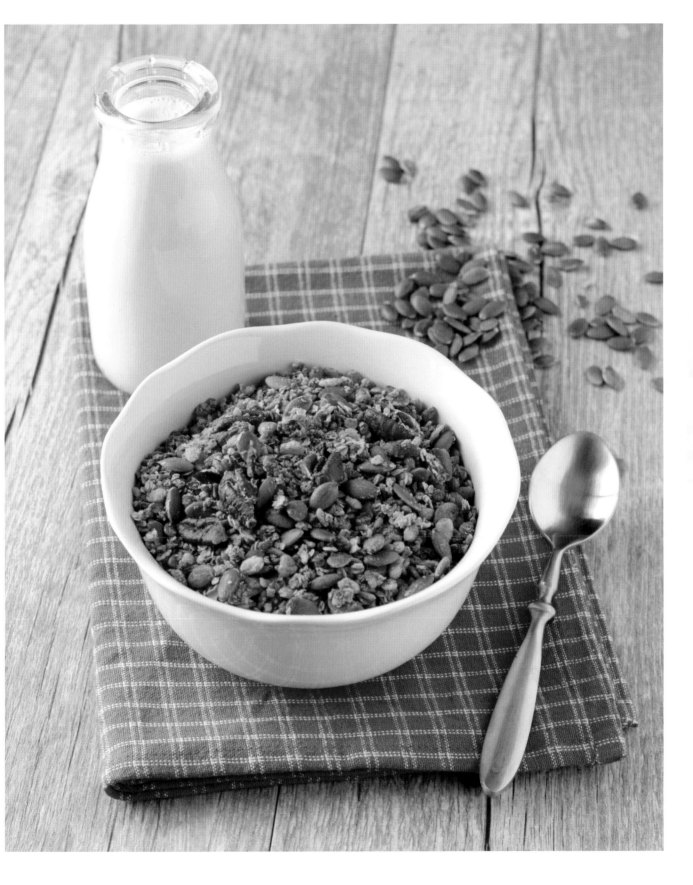

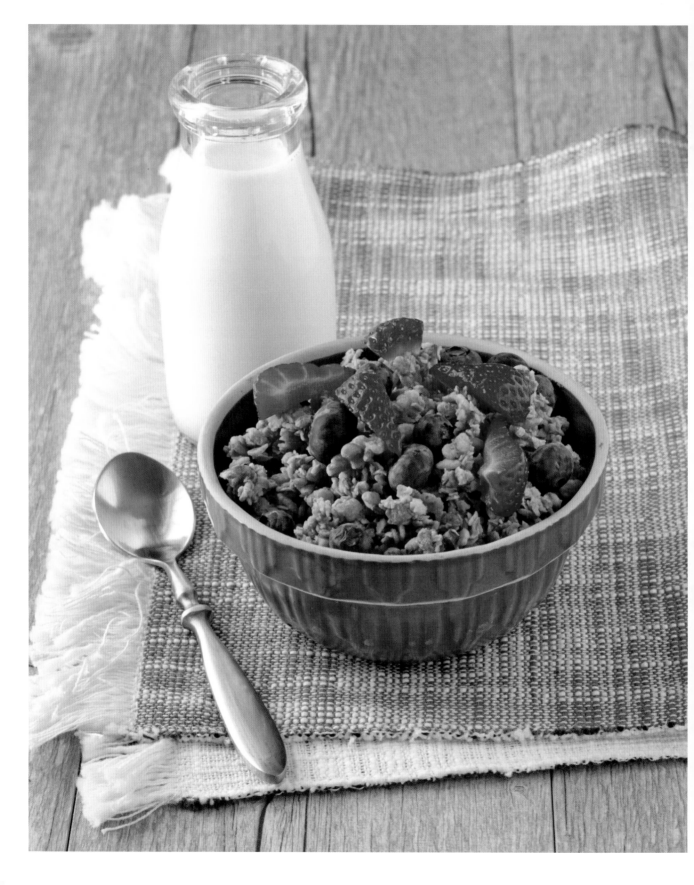

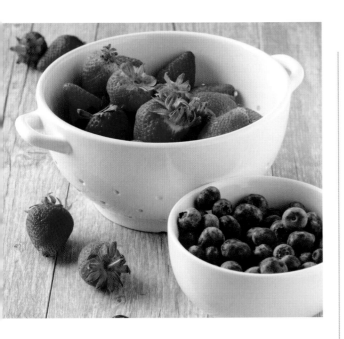

VERY BERRY GRANOLA

YIELD: 6 SERVINGS, ¾ CUP (75 G) EACH

My husband loves my homemade granola and cereal and eats it nearly every day. This is one of his favorites: a delicious concoction that's slowly baked until it's super-crunchy and infused with berry flavor. For an extra hit of berry goodness, top it with fresh strawberries and blueberries. As with the Pumpkin Pecan Granola on page 46, stick to the suggested serving size so you don't overdose on oats, which have moderate levels of FODMAPs.

2 CUPS (64 G) GLUTEN-FREE CRISPY RICE CEREAL (SUCH AS EREWHON—CHECK PRODUCT INGREDIENTS FOR FODMAPS)

1½ CUPS (120 G) QUICK-COOKING OATS (GLUTEN-FREE IF NECESSARY)

½ CUP (60 G) CHOPPED WALNUTS

⅓ CUP (80 ML) WATER

⅓ CUP (67 G) SUGAR

¼ TEASPOON SALT

2 TABLESPOONS (28 ML) WALNUT OIL

1 TABLESPOON (15 ML) RASPBERRY EXTRACT (IMITATION IS FINE)

Preheat the oven to 300°F (150°C, or gas mark 2). Line a large rimmed baking sheet with parchment paper. In a large bowl, mix together the rice cereal, oats, and walnuts.

Combine the water, sugar, and salt in a small saucepan over medium heat. Cook and stir until the sugar is dissolved. Remove the mixture from the heat. Stir in the walnut oil and raspberry extract. Pour into the oat mixture and stir until thoroughly combined.

Spread the mixture on the prepared baking sheet and bake for about 50 to 60 minutes or until dry and lightly toasted. Do not stir during the baking time! Let cool before breaking apart into chunks. Store in an airtight container for several weeks.

PEANUT BUTTER OVERNIGHT QUINOA AND OATS

YIELD: 2 SERVINGS

Warm porridge is just the ticket on winter mornings, but in summer, I usually crave something cooler. Enter this overnight oats recipe! To keep the recipe low-FODMAP, I replaced half of the oats with quinoa flakes, which are generally more tolerable. I admit it: Sometimes I don't care for the slightly bitter taste of quinoa flakes, but I don't notice it at all in this flavorful recipe. I use powdered peanut butter here because it's so much lower in fat, but regular peanut butter will work fine, too. And the chia seeds help make the mixture pleasantly thick and creamy.

½ CUP (40 G) QUICK-COOKING OATS (GLUTEN-FREE IF NECESSARY)

½ CUP (51 G) QUINOA FLAKES

2 TABLESPOONS (26 G) GROUND CHIA SEEDS

¼ CUP (24 G) POWDERED PEANUT BUTTER (OR 2 TABLESPOONS, 32 G, NATURAL CREAMY PEANUT BUTTER)

1¼ CUPS (285 ML) LACTOSE-FREE OR NONDAIRY MILK

1 TABLESPOON (15 ML) PURE MAPLE SYRUP

¼ TEASPOON PURE VANILLA EXTRACT

2 TEASPOONS MINI SEMISWEET CHOCOLATE CHIPS OR FINELY CHOPPED DARK CHOCOLATE IF TOLERATED (OPTIONAL)

Combine the oats, quinoa flakes, chia seeds, and powdered peanut butter in a bowl or a container with a lid. Pour in the milk, maple syrup, and vanilla. Stir well. Cover with the lid and refrigerate overnight. In the morning, stir in the chocolate chips and enjoy immediately.

Make it vegan! Use canned light coconut milk or other nondairy milk and use tolerable vegan chocolate in place of regular.

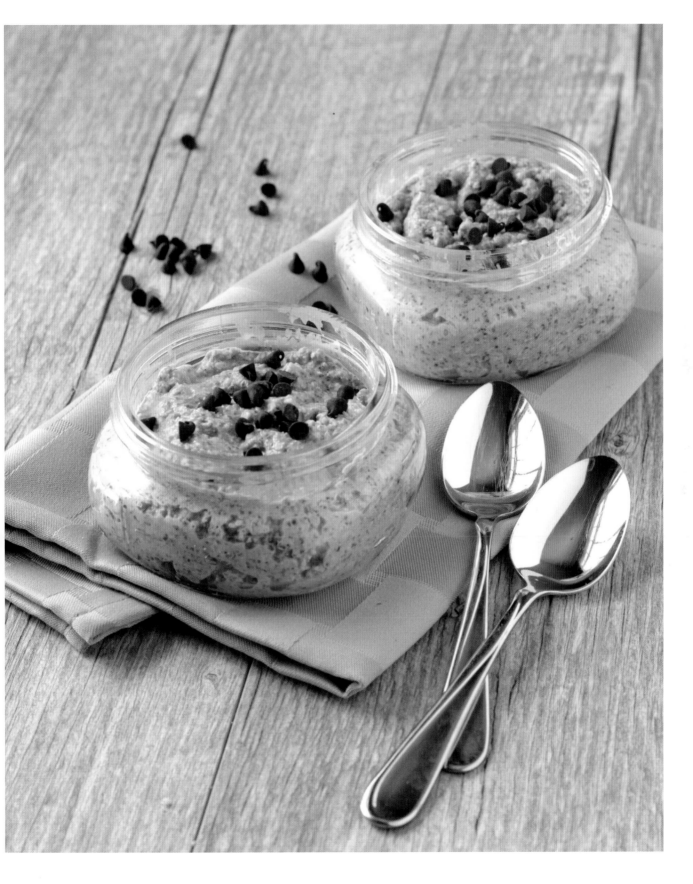

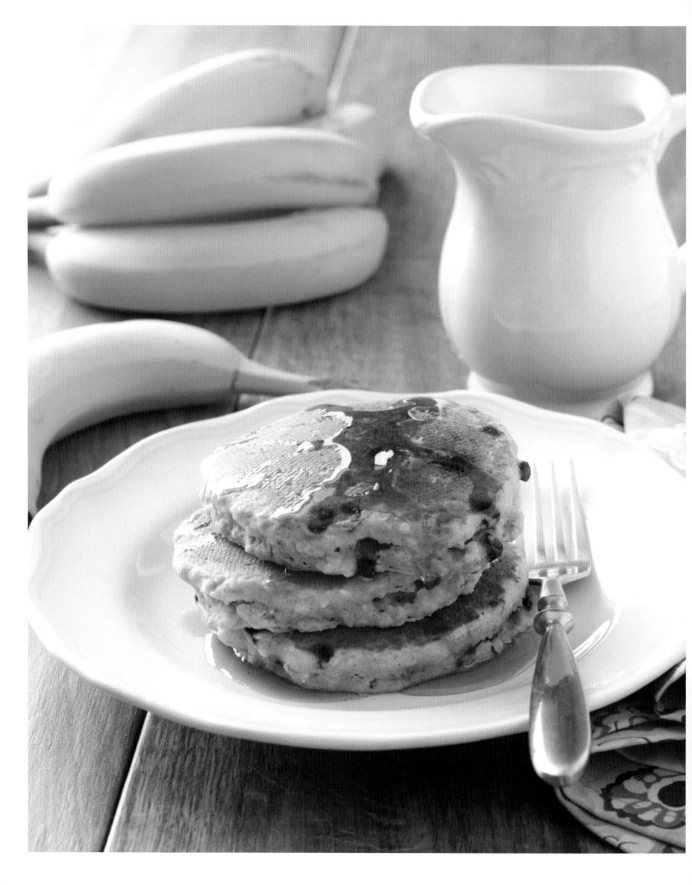

BANANA OATMEAL PANCAKES

YIELD: 10 PANCAKES

Do you ever end up with a single lonely banana lingering in your fruit bowl at the end of the week? Don't throw it away: Pair it with oatmeal and make these healthy, filling pancakes instead! All they need is a light drizzle of pure maple syrup—plus some chocolate for a decadent finishing touch. And they're so easy to pull together on a busy Saturday morning.

½ CUP (113 G) MASHED RIPE BANANA (ABOUT 1 LARGE)

1¼ CUPS (285 ML) LACTOSE-FREE OR NONDAIRY MILK, DIVIDED

1 TABLESPOON (15 ML) CANOLA OIL OR OTHER NEUTRAL OIL

1 CUP (80 G) QUICK-COOKING OATS (GLUTEN-FREE IF NECESSARY)

1 CUP (162 G) BASIC FLOUR BLEND (PAGE 38)

1 TABLESPOON (14 G) BAKING POWDER

1 TEASPOON SUGAR

½ TEASPOON GROUND CINNAMON

¼ TEASPOON SALT

2 TABLESPOONS (22 G) FINELY CHOPPED DARK CHOCOLATE (OR MINI SEMISWEET CHOCOLATE CHIPS, IF TOLERATED)

Heat an electric griddle to 375°F (190°C) or a stovetop griddle over medium heat. In a large bowl, combine the mashed banana, 1 cup (235 ml) of the milk, canola oil, and oats. Let the mixture sit for 5 to 10 minutes, allowing the oats to soak up the liquid. Then stir in the Basic Flour Blend, baking powder, sugar, cinnamon, and salt. Stir in the remaining ¼ cup (60 ml) milk and the chopped dark chocolate. Add more milk, if necessary, to bring the batter to a pourable consistency.

For each pancake, pour ¼ cup (60 ml) batter onto the griddle. Flip after a few minutes, when the bottom edges start to look dry. Cook until golden brown on the other side. Repeat with the remaining batter.

Make it vegan! Use canned coconut or other nondairy milk instead of lactose-free dairy milk and use a tolerable vegan chocolate in place of regular.

FLUFFY BLUEBERRY PANCAKES

YIELD: 8 PANCAKES

These are quite possibly the best pancakes I've had, gluten-free or otherwise! They're so moist and fluffy that they don't really need syrup—although I always drizzle a little bit of maple syrup over mine anyway. And no specialty ingredients are required, either: Souring the milk with vinegar or lemon juice makes a quick lactose-free buttermilk substitute. And it's simple to make a vegan version of these pancakes, too. What's not to like?

1 CUP (235 ML) LACTOSE-FREE OR NONDAIRY MILK (SUCH AS CANNED COCONUT MILK)

1 TABLESPOON (15 ML) VINEGAR OR FRESH LEMON JUICE

1 ½ CUPS (243 G) BASIC FLOUR BLEND (PAGE 38)

2 TABLESPOONS (26 G) SUGAR

2 TEASPOONS BAKING POWDER

½ TEASPOON SALT

1 LARGE EGG

2 TABLESPOONS (28 G) MELTED UNSALTED BUTTER, VIRGIN COCONUT OIL, OR VEGAN MARGARINE

½ CUP (75 G) FRESH BLUEBERRIES

Heat a electric griddle to 375°F (190°C) or a stovetop griddle over medium heat. Measure out the milk in a glass measuring cup and stir in the vinegar. Set aside to sour for 5 to 10 minutes.

Combine the Basic Flour Blend, sugar, baking powder, and salt in a large bowl. In a medium bowl, lightly beat the egg. Whisk in the soured milk. Slowly pour in the melted butter while whisking. Pour the egg mixture into the flour mixture and stir until there are no lumps. Fold in the blueberries.

Grease the griddle, if necessary. Pour about ¼ cup (60 ml) batter onto the griddle for each pancake. Cook for a few minutes until bubbles form on top and then flip. Continue to cook until the other side is golden brown. Repeat with the remaining batter.

Make it vegan! Use the vegan suggestions for the milk and melted butter and replace the egg with 1 tablespoon (15 ml) nondairy milk plus ½ teaspoon baking powder.

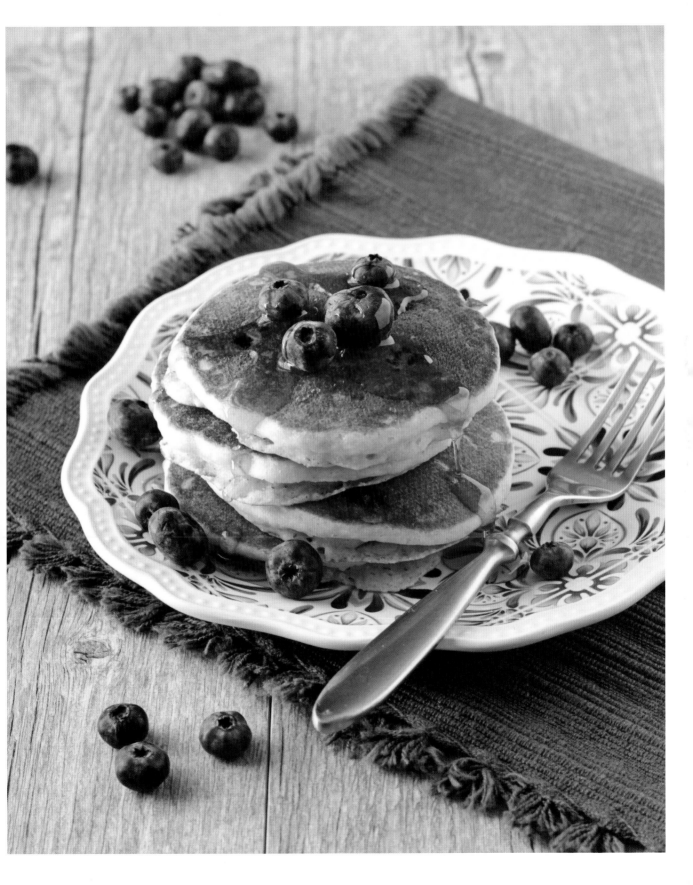

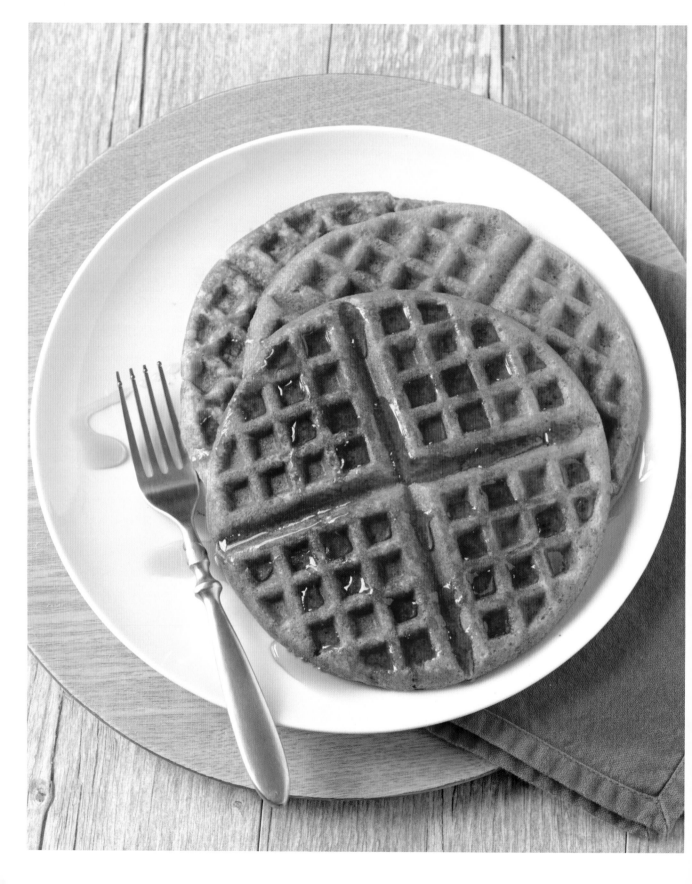

PUMPKIN SPICE WAFFLES

YIELD: 4 WAFFLES, 8 INCHES (20 CM) EACH

Nothing says fall like the combination of pumpkin and aromatic baking spices such as cinnamon, nutmeg, and cloves. These spice-laden waffles are guaranteed to warm you up from the inside out. Crisp on the outside and tender and fluffy on the inside, they're fabulous on a chilly weekend morning.

1½ CUPS (355 ML) LACTOSE-FREE OR NONDAIRY MILK

1 TABLESPOON (15 ML) FRESH LEMON JUICE

1⅔ CUPS (270 G) BASIC FLOUR BLEND (PAGE 38)

1 TABLESPOON (15 G) BROWN SUGAR

2 TEASPOONS BAKING POWDER

½ TEASPOON SALT

1½ TEASPOONS GROUND CINNAMON

½ TEASPOON GROUND GINGER

¼ TEASPOON GROUND NUTMEG

⅛ TEASPOON GROUND CLOVES

½ CUP (123 G) PUMPKIN PUREE

2 TABLESPOONS (28 ML) CANOLA OIL OR OTHER NEUTRAL OIL

Turn on the waffle iron to preheat. Blend together the milk and lemon juice in a medium bowl and let sit for 5 to 10 minutes to sour.

Meanwhile, in a large bowl, combine the Basic Flour Blend, brown sugar, baking powder, salt, cinnamon, ginger, nutmeg, and ground cloves. Stir the pumpkin puree and canola oil into the milk mixture. Slowly add the milk-pumpkin mixture to the flour mixture, stirring to prevent lumps. Stir until well blended and smooth.

Spray the waffle iron with cooking spray, if necessary, and pour the batter into the iron according to manufacturer's instructions. (I have an 8-inch [20 cm] round waffle iron and use about ⅔ cup [160 ml] of batter per waffle). Close the waffle iron and cook until the iron stops steaming, about 3 to 5 minutes or according to the instructions. Remove the waffle with a fork and serve immediately.

Make it vegan! It couldn't be simpler: Just use nondairy milk.

BANANA BREAD BROWN RICE PORRIDGE

YIELD: 2 SERVINGS

This is a great wintertime breakfast, and you'll love it, too, especially if you're a banana bread fiend. It'll keep you going all morning long, and it's so warm and comforting. Rice makes a wonderful porridge, and it reminds me of rice pudding, one of my favorite desserts. Plus, it's healthier than it tastes: The brown rice lends it a hefty dose of fiber. If you don't have much time in the morning, you can make it the night before and reheat it in the microwave before you rush out the door.

1 MEDIUM BANANA, MASHED

2 CUPS (475 ML) WATER

1 CUP (235 ML) LIGHT CANNED COCONUT MILK (OR LACTOSE-FREE COW'S MILK)

½ CUP (95 G) BROWN RICE

1 TABLESPOON (15 G) BROWN SUGAR

1 TEASPOON PURE VANILLA EXTRACT

PINCH OF SALT

½ TEASPOON GROUND CINNAMON

2 TABLESPOONS (15 G) CHOPPED TOASTED WALNUTS

Combine the mashed banana, water, and coconut milk in a large saucepan. Stir in the brown rice, brown sugar, vanilla, and salt. Bring to a boil. Reduce the heat and simmer, uncovered, stirring frequently, for 30 to 40 minutes, until most of the liquid is absorbed and the rice is tender. Stir in the cinnamon and serve with the chopped walnuts sprinkled on top.

POTATO FRITTATA, TWO WAYS

YIELD: 4 SERVINGS

Light yet filling, these frittatas make an excellent breakfast or brunch, and they're great for dinner, too. They're already a breeze to make, but to make life even easier, you can use thawed frozen hash browns in place of the shredded potatoes (just be sure to check the ingredients list for FODMAPs). Serve them at breakfast with Mom's Best Biscuits on page 76, or try them as an evening meal with a tossed salad.

6 LARGE EGGS

¼ CUP (60 ML) LACTOSE-FREE OR NONDAIRY MILK

¾ TEASPOON KOSHER SALT

½ TEASPOON FRESHLY GROUND BLACK PEPPER

1 TABLESPOON (15 ML) OLIVE OIL

2 CUPS (220 G) SHREDDED POTATOES

Preheat the oven to 350°F (180°C, or gas mark 4). In a large bowl, whisk together the eggs, milk, kosher salt, black pepper, and any add-in ingredients (see below).

Heat the olive oil in a 10-inch (25.5 cm) ovenproof skillet (cast iron or nonstick works best) over medium-high heat. Add the shredded potatoes and sauté until browned, about 8 to 10 minutes. Remove from the heat and pour the egg mixture evenly over the potatoes. Place the skillet in the oven and bake for 20 to 25 minutes until puffed up and very lightly browned. Cut into wedges and serve. Store leftovers in the refrigerator for up to 2 days.

PESTO POTATO FRITTATA

To the egg mixture, stir in: ¼ cup (60 ml) Spinach Basil Pesto (page 41) and ½ cup (50 g) grated Parmesan cheese.

SPINACH AND SWISS POTATO FRITTATA

To the egg mixture, stir in: 2 cups (60 g) fresh baby spinach, chopped; 4 scallions, sliced (green part only); and ½ cup (55 g) shredded Swiss cheese.

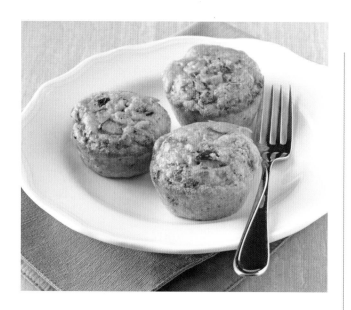

ZUCCHINI QUINOA EGG MUFFINS

YIELD: 6 MUFFINS

These savory muffins are the perfect blend of protein and carbs, and they're sure to keep your belly happy until lunchtime. Dig out your muffin pan from the back of the cupboard and make a batch this weekend. Then heat them up for a quick, savory breakfast on weekday mornings.

1 TABLESPOON (15 ML) OLIVE OIL

1 CUP (120 G) DICED ZUCCHINI

¼ CUP (38 G) DICED RED BELL PEPPER

5 LARGE EGGS

¾ CUP (139 G) COOKED QUINOA

3 TABLESPOONS (15 G) GRATED PARMESAN CHEESE

2 SCALLIONS (GREEN PARTS ONLY), THINLY SLICED

1 TEASPOON ITALIAN HERB SEASONING (PAGE 40)

½ TEASPOON KOSHER SALT

¼ TEASPOON FRESHLY GROUND BLACK PEPPER

Preheat the oven to 325°F (160°C, or gas mark 3). Spray 6 of the cups in a muffin pan with olive oil cooking spray.

Heat the olive oil in a medium skillet over medium heat. Sauté the zucchini and red bell pepper until lightly browned and tender, about 10 to 12 minutes. In a large bowl, beat the eggs. Stir in the cooked zucchini mixture, quinoa, Parmesan cheese, scallions, Italian herb seasoning, kosher salt, and black pepper.

Divide the mixture evenly among the prepared muffin cups and bake for 20 minutes until golden on top. Cool slightly before removing from the pan. Enjoy immediately or store in the refrigerator for up to 4 days or the freezer for up to 3 months.

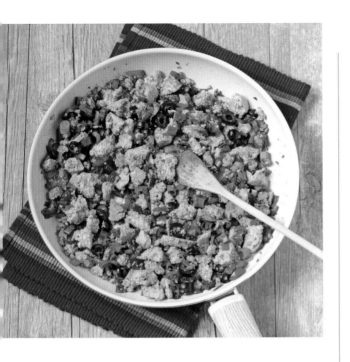

TOFU SCRAMBLE RANCHEROS

YIELD: 4 SERVINGS

If you're in the market for a tasty vegan alternative to scrambled eggs, look no further. The turmeric gives the tofu a yellow hue, making it look just like eggs, and it's just as protein-rich and satisfying as eggs are, too. Enjoy this dish in the morning with low-FODMAP toast or for lunch or dinner with a side of rice. Oh, and since ancho chile pepper hasn't yet been tested for FODMAPs, only use it if you know you can tolerate it (the scramble will still taste amazing without the chile—trust me!).

1 TABLESPOON (15 ML) OLIVE OIL

½ CUP (75 G) CHOPPED GREEN BELL PEPPER

½ CUP (90 G) CHOPPED TOMATO

1 CAN (2.25 OUNCES, OR 62 G) SLICED BLACK OLIVES, DRAINED

1 TEASPOON KOSHER SALT

½ TEASPOON FRESHLY GROUND BLACK PEPPER

½ TEASPOON GROUND CUMIN

¼ TEASPOON ANCHO CHILE POWDER (OPTIONAL)

2 CUPS (496 G) DRAINED, CRUMBLED EXTRA-FIRM TOFU

½ TEASPOON GROUND TURMERIC

2 SCALLIONS (GREENS PART ONLY), SLICED

¼ CUP (4 G) CHOPPED FRESH CILANTRO

Heat the olive oil in a large skillet over medium-high heat. Add the green bell pepper and sauté until tender, about 3 to 4 minutes. Reduce the heat to medium-low and stir in the tomato, black olives, kosher salt, black pepper, cumin, and ancho chile powder.

Add the tofu to the skillet and sprinkle with the turmeric. Cook, stirring gently, until the tofu turns yellow and is heated through, about 5 minutes. Stir in the sliced scallions and chopped fresh cilantro and serve immediately.

BANANA BREAD

YIELD: 1 LOAF (ABOUT 12 SLICES)

Who doesn't love banana bread? It's always been one of my favorite treats, that's for sure. So I came up with this low-FODMAP version, which can also be made vegan by substituting the Chia Egg Replacer on page 39 for the egg. And I've replaced a portion of the flour with plain tapioca flour, which gives the bread extra elasticity and moistness. The coconut oil does add another subtle layer of flavor, but if you haven't got it on hand, you could always use melted butter instead.

1 CUP (162 G) BASIC FLOUR BLEND (PAGE 38)

⅓ CUP (40 G) TAPIOCA FLOUR

½ CUP (100 G) SUGAR

1 TEASPOON GROUND CINNAMON

½ TEASPOON SALT

½ TEASPOON BAKING SODA

1 CUP (225 G) MASHED BANANAS (ABOUT 2 LARGE)

¼ CUP (56 G) VIRGIN COCONUT OIL, MELTED

1 LARGE EGG OR 1 CHIA EGG REPLACER (PAGE 39)

1 TEASPOON PURE VANILLA EXTRACT

Preheat the oven to 325°F (160°C, or gas mark 3). Lightly spray a 4 x 8-inch (10 x 20 cm) loaf pan with cooking spray.

In a medium bowl, combine the Basic Flour Blend, tapioca flour, sugar, cinnamon, salt, and baking soda. In a large bowl, stir together the mashed bananas, melted coconut oil, egg, and vanilla. Add the flour mixture and stir until well combined.

Pour the batter into the prepared loaf pan. Bake for 50 to 60 minutes until a toothpick inserted in the middle comes out clean and the top springs back when lightly touched. Let the banana bread cool in the pan for 5 to 10 minutes before turning it out onto a wire rack and slicing.

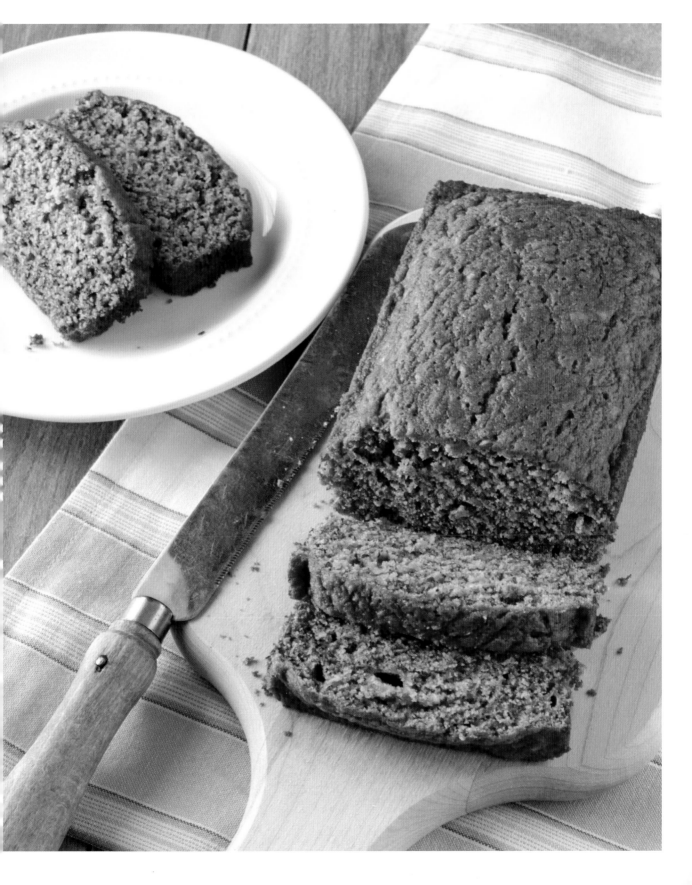

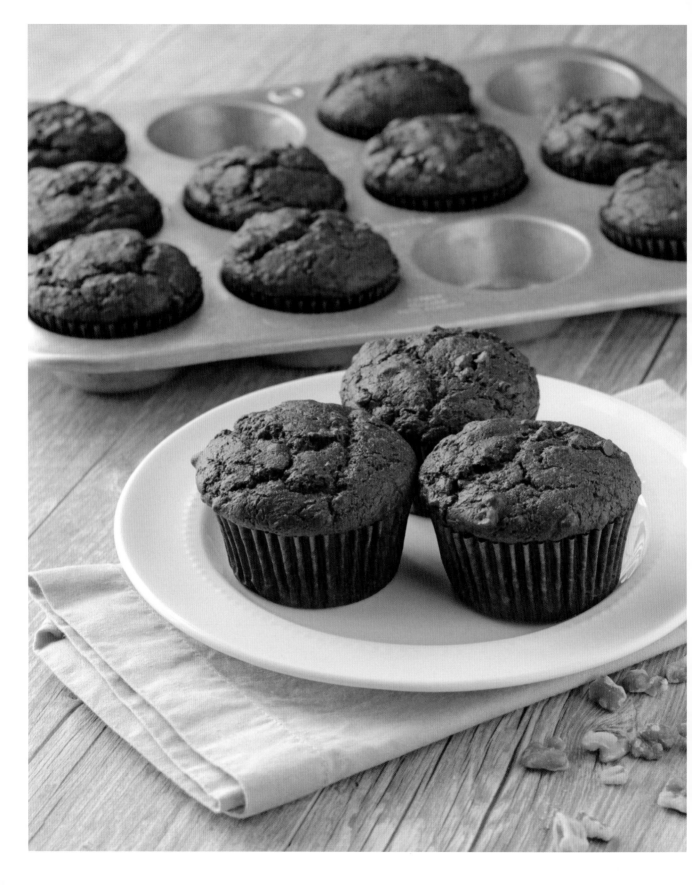

DOUBLE CHOCOLATE BANANA MUFFINS

YIELD: 12 MUFFINS

Chocolate and banana is one of the world's great flavor combinations, and these muffins prove it. My husband and I love them, so I always have a batch or two tucked away in the freezer. They're the ideal mid-morning snack: reach for one when you're pouring that second cup of coffee or tea.

1½ CUPS (243 G) BASIC FLOUR BLEND (PAGE 38)

½ CUP (100 G) SUGAR

⅓ CUP (30 G) UNSWEETENED COCOA POWDER

2 TEASPOONS BAKING POWDER

½ TEASPOON SALT

1 CUP (225 G) MASHED BANANAS

1 LARGE EGG

⅓ CUP (80 ML) CANOLA OIL OR OTHER NEUTRAL OIL

¼ CUP (60 ML) LACTOSE-FREE OR NONDAIRY MILK

1 TEASPOON PURE VANILLA EXTRACT

½ CUP (85 G) CHOPPED DARK CHOCOLATE (OR MINI SEMISWEET CHOCOLATE CHIPS, IF TOLERATED)

½ CUP (60 G) FINELY CHOPPED WALNUTS

Preheat the oven to 350°F (180°C, or gas mark 4). Line or grease a standard-size 12-cup muffin pan.

In a medium bowl, stir together the Basic Flour Blend, sugar, cocoa powder, baking powder, and salt. In a large bowl, combine the mashed bananas, egg, canola oil, milk, and vanilla. Add the flour mixture, chopped dark chocolate, and walnuts. Stir until well blended.

Fill each muffin cup two-thirds to three-quarters full with batter. Bake for 18 to 20 minutes until a toothpick inserted in the middle of a muffin comes out clean and the muffin tops spring back when lightly touched. Let the muffins cool in the pan before turning them out onto a wire rack. Store in an airtight container for several days or freeze for up to 3 months.

Make it vegan! Replace the egg with a Chia Egg Replacer (page 39) plus an extra ½ teaspoon baking powder; use nondairy milk and tolerable vegan chocolate.

CRANBERRY ORANGE SCONES

YIELD: 12 SCONES

These low-FODMAP scones make an ideal breakfast—especially during the holiday season, when they're great companions for a cup of coffee or green tea. Go ahead and use frozen cranberries in this recipe, but be sure to keep them frozen until you add them to the dough: If you let them thaw before using them, their juices will turn the dough pink! To avoid this, I chop the frozen cranberries and then stick them back in the freezer until the last minute. And don't skip the final steps. Brushing these scones with milk and finishing them with a sprinkle of sugar really makes them shine.

1¾ CUPS (284 G) BASIC FLOUR BLEND (PAGE 38)

½ CUP (60 G) TAPIOCA FLOUR

⅓ CUP (67 G) SUGAR, PLUS MORE FOR SPRINKLING ON TOP

2 TEASPOONS BAKING POWDER

1 TEASPOON GRATED ORANGE ZEST

½ TEASPOON SALT

5 TABLESPOONS (70 G) UNSALTED BUTTER, CUT INTO PIECES AND CHILLED

½ CUP (55 G) COARSELY CHOPPED FRESH OR FROZEN CRANBERRIES

⅔ CUP (160 ML) LACTOSE-FREE LOW-FAT MILK, PLUS MORE FOR BRUSHING ON TOP

Preheat the oven to 400°F (200°C, or gas mark 6). Line a large baking sheet with parchment paper.

In a large bowl, combine the Basic Flour Blend, tapioca flour, sugar, baking powder, orange zest, and salt. Using a fork or a pastry blender, cut in the butter until the mixture resembles coarse meal. Stir in the cranberries. Add the milk and mix until a dough forms.

Lightly flour a work surface and using floured hands, divide the dough into two pieces. Place each portion of dough onto the floured work surface and shape into a 5-inch (13 cm) diameter round disk. Cut each disk into 6 slices (like a pizza). Transfer to the prepared baking sheet. Lightly brush each scone with milk and sprinkle with sugar.

Bake for 10 to 12 minutes until golden brown. Let cool on the baking sheet for 5 minutes before transferring to a wire rack.

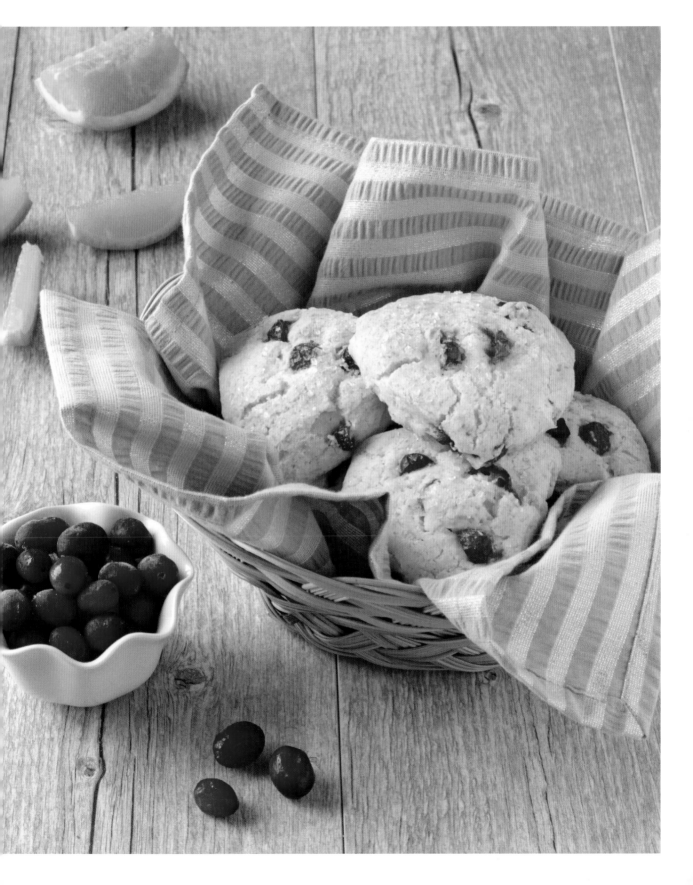

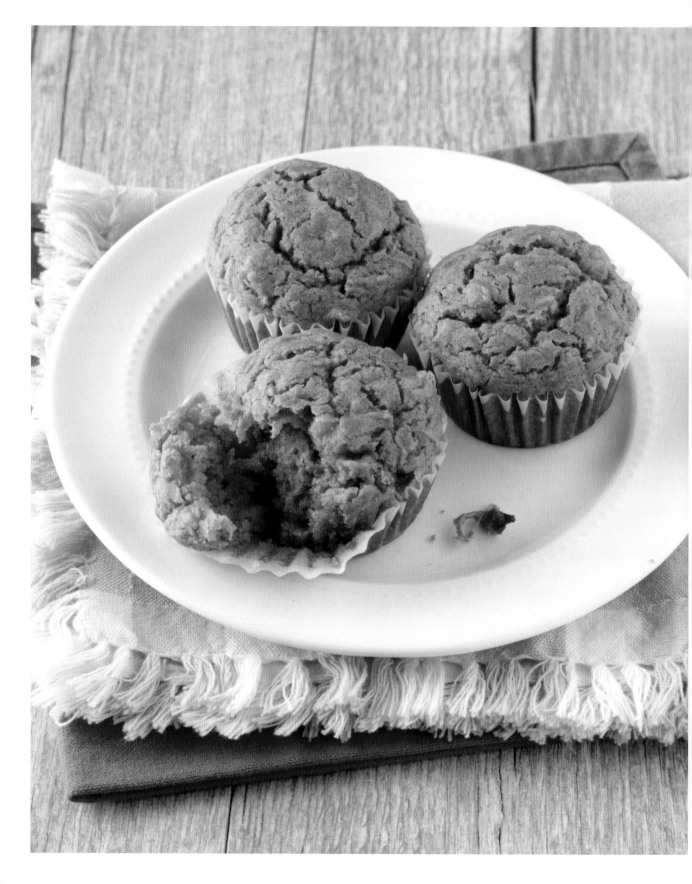

QUINOA MORNING GLORY MUFFINS

YIELD: 12 MUFFINS

Carrots, pineapple, and quinoa join forces in these spiced muffins to make a wholesome, filling breakfast. I know quinoa flour has a strong scent and flavor that some folks find off-putting, but toasting the flour before using it smoothes out its bitterness and lends it a nice nutty flavor. Plus, quinoa flour is packed with fiber and protein, making it an excellent low-FODMAP choice. While fresh pineapple has been tested as low-FODMAP, canned pineapple in juice has not been tested, so ask your dietitian if this is an appropriate recipe for you.

1⅓ CUPS (149 G) QUINOA FLOUR

½ CUP (60 G) CHOPPED WALNUTS

⅔ CUP (80 G) TAPIOCA FLOUR

2 TEASPOONS BAKING POWDER

1 TEASPOON GROUND CINNAMON

½ TEASPOON SALT

1 LARGE EGG

⅔ CUP (150 G) PACKED BROWN SUGAR

⅓ CUP (80 ML) CANOLA OIL OR OTHER NEUTRAL OIL

1 CAN (8 OUNCES, OR 225 G) CRUSHED PINEAPPLE IN JUICE (UNDRAINED)

1 CUP (110 G) FINELY SHREDDED CARROTS

¼ CUP (60 ML) LACTOSE-FREE MILK

1 TEASPOON PURE VANILLA EXTRACT

Preheat the oven to 350°F (180°C, or gas mark 4). Line or grease a standard-size 12-cup muffin pan.

In a small dry skillet, heat the quinoa flour over medium heat. Cook and stir until the flour is toasted: It should emit a nutty scent and turn light brown. Transfer the quinoa flour to a large bowl and let cool. In the same dry skillet, toast the walnuts over medium heat until lightly browned. Remove the walnuts from the skillet and set aside to cool.

To the bowl with the quinoa flour, add the tapioca flour, baking powder, cinnamon, and salt and combine.

In a large bowl, lightly beat the egg. Stir in the brown sugar, canola oil, crushed pineapple, shredded carrots, milk, and vanilla. Add to the flour mixture and blend well. Stir in the toasted walnuts.

Fill each muffin cup about two-thirds full with batter. Bake for 20 to 22 minutes until a toothpick inserted in the middle of a muffin comes out clean. Store in an airtight container for 3 to 4 days or freeze for up to 3 months.

Make it vegan! Use a Chia Egg Replacer (page 39) plus an extra ½ teaspoon baking powder instead of a regular egg and use nondairy milk.

LEMON BLUEBERRY BAKED DOUGHNUTS

YIELD: 12 DOUGHNUTS

Even if you're not on a low-FODMAP eating plan, fat- and sugar-laden store-bought doughnuts aren't usually a healthy breakfast choice. That's where these homemade baked doughnuts come in. They're both low-FODMAP and a lot lower in fat than regular doughnuts. Lemon and blueberry are a natural flavor match, and the lemon glaze brings a nice balance of tartness and sweetness. This recipe was inspired by *Parade* magazine.

2 LARGE EGGS

½ CUP (120 ML) LACTOSE-FREE MILK

⅔ CUP (133 G) GRANULATED SUGAR

4 TABLESPOONS (55 G) UNSALTED BUTTER, MELTED

½ TEASPOON GRATED LEMON ZEST

2 CUPS (324 G) BASIC FLOUR BLEND (PAGE 38)

1½ TEASPOONS BAKING POWDER

½ TEASPOON SALT

¾ CUP (109 G) FRESH BLUEBERRIES

1½ CUPS (180 G) CONFECTIONERS' SUGAR, SIFTED

¼ CUP (60 ML) FRESH LEMON JUICE

Preheat the oven to 350°F (180°C, or gas mark 4). Coat a 12-cavity doughnut pan (or two 6-cavity pans) with cooking spray.

In a large bowl, lightly beat the eggs. Stir in the milk, granulated sugar, melted butter, and lemon zest. In a medium bowl, stir together the Basic Flour Blend, baking powder, and salt. Add to the butter mixture and beat until well combined. Fold in the blueberries.

Fill each doughnut cup about two-thirds full with batter. Bake for 12 to 14 minutes until just starting to brown lightly on the edges and a toothpick inserted into a doughnut comes out clean. Let cool in the pan for about 10 minutes before transferring the doughnuts to a wire rack.

To make the glaze, stir together the confectioners' sugar and lemon juice until smooth and free from lumps. Place a sheet of waxed paper under the cooling rack. Dip the top of each doughnut into the glaze and place back on the cooling rack to dry (and to allow the excess glaze to drip off). Store in an airtight container for 2 to 3 days.

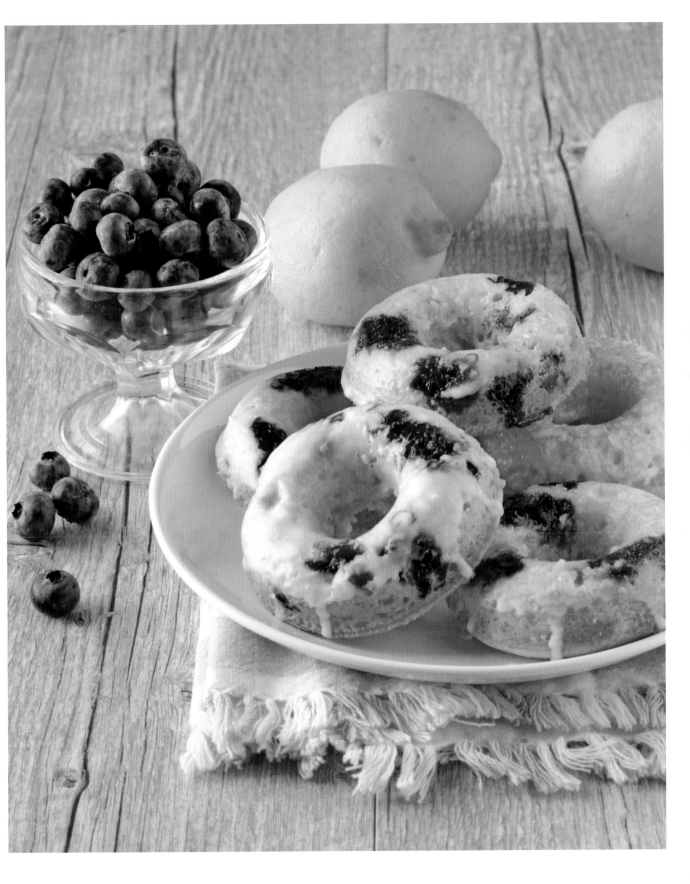

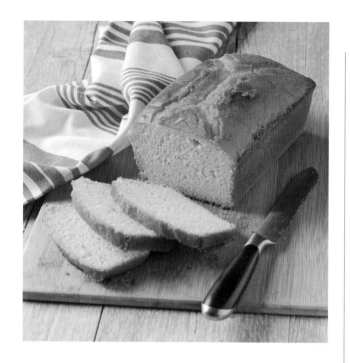

SANDWICH BREAD

YIELD: 1 LOAF

Baking gluten-free breads can be tricky—especially when you're avoiding gums, like xanthan gum—but I've figured out a couple ways to ensure a good result every time. First, proofing the yeast by combining it with sugar before adding warm water is a good idea. It will form a foamy head, which shows that the yeast is active. Also, adding a few tablespoons (30 g) of sweet white rice flour, or glutinous rice flour, to the mix helps the dough rise and improves its elasticity. (Despite its name, glutinous rice flour is gluten-free.) Perfect for toast and sandwiches, this bread also makes great bread crumbs (see page 73).

1 TABLESPOON (12 G) ACTIVE DRY YEAST

4 TABLESPOONS (50 G) GRANULATED SUGAR, DIVIDED

1¼ CUPS (285 ML) WARM WATER (110°F, OR 43°C)

2¼ CUPS (365 G) BASIC FLOUR BLEND (PAGE 38)

¾ CUP (90 G) TAPIOCA FLOUR

3 TABLESPOONS (30 G) SWEET WHITE RICE FLOUR (ALSO CALLED GLUTINOUS RICE FLOUR)

1½ TEASPOONS SALT

1 TEASPOON BAKING POWDER

¼ CUP (60 ML) CANOLA OIL OR OTHER NEUTRAL OIL

2 LARGE EGGS, LIGHTLY BEATEN

2 TEASPOONS VINEGAR

1 TABLESPOON (15 ML) OLIVE OIL OR MELTED UNSALTED BUTTER

Preheat the oven to 375°F (190°C, or gas mark 5). Spray a 4 x 8-inch (10 x 20 cm) loaf pan with cooking spray.

Proof the yeast by combining it with 1 tablespoon (13 g) of the sugar in a medium bowl and slowly stirring in the warm water. Let the mixture sit until a foamy head develops, about 5 to 10 minutes.

Meanwhile, combine the Basic Flour Blend, tapioca flour, sweet rice flour, remaining 3 tablespoons (39 g) sugar, salt, and baking powder in a large bowl attached to a stand mixer. Mix on low speed until the dry ingredients are combined. Add the yeast mixture, canola oil, eggs, and vinegar. Mix on low speed until just combined. Scrape down the sides of the bowl and then beat on medium speed for 3 minutes. (The mixture will look more like a thin cake batter than a dough.) Pour into the prepared pan.

Let the dough rise in a warm enclosed space—such as a microwave, with a cup of hot water placed next to it—for 20 to 25 minutes until the batter has risen just up to the rim of the baking pan, but no more: Otherwise, it might overflow when baking! (Note: If the environment is not warm enough, the dough may take longer to rise.)

Immediately place the pan in the oven and bake for 45 to 50 minutes until the bread is well browned on top. Remove from the oven and brush with the olive oil. Let cool completely before removing from the pan and slicing. Like most gluten-free breads, this bread is best enjoyed within a day or two, so if you won't use it all right away, freeze it and thaw slices as needed.

Bread crumbs. Preheat the oven to 300°F (150°C, or gas mark 2). Lay bread slices out on a large rimmed baking sheet. Bake for 10 minutes and then flip and bake 10 minutes more or until the bread is dried out. (Note that baking times may vary depending on the type or brand of bread used.) Remove from the oven and let cool. Grind the bread in a food processor until you've achieved the desired crumb size. Homemade bread crumbs keep well in the freezer, and there's no need to thaw them before using.

MULTIGRAIN VEGAN ENGLISH MUFFINS

YIELD: 6 ENGLISH MUFFINS

These five-grain English muffins are a handy bread option if you're vegan or if you don't tolerate eggs. But non-vegans are sure to love them, too—either toasted for breakfast, as a hamburger bun, or as part of a sandwich for lunch. You can buy oat flour pre-ground, or you can grind it yourself in a clean coffee grinder or food processor. And I usually use plain corn flour instead of masa harina, which tastes vaguely like fresh lime. Because the dough is so thin, it's best to bake them in small ramekins, which are just the right size.

2¼ TEASPOONS (ONE 0.25-OUNCE PACKET, OR 9 G) ACTIVE DRY YEAST

1 TABLESPOON (13 G) SUGAR

1⅓ CUPS (315 ML) WARM WATER (110°F, OR 43°C)

⅔ CUP (107 G) BROWN RICE FLOUR

⅔ CUP (80 G) TAPIOCA FLOUR

½ CUP (70 G) OAT FLOUR (GLUTEN-FREE IF NECESSARY)

¼ CUP (29 G) CORN FLOUR

¼ CUP (28 G) QUINOA FLOUR, TOASTED IF DESIRED

2 TABLESPOONS (20 G) SWEET WHITE RICE FLOUR

2 TABLESPOONS (26 G) GROUND CHIA SEEDS

1½ TEASPOONS BAKING POWDER

½ TEASPOON SALT

1 TABLESPOON (15 ML) CANOLA OIL OR OTHER NEUTRAL OIL

1 TEASPOON VINEGAR

Preheat the oven to 375°F (190°C, or gas mark 5). Spray six 4-inch (10 cm) ramekins generously with cooking spray.

Proof the yeast by combing it with the sugar in a medium bowl and slowly stirring in the warm water. Let the mixture sit until a foamy head develops, about 5 to 10 minutes.

Meanwhile, combine the brown rice flour, tapioca flour, oat flour, corn flour, quinoa flour, sweet white rice flour, ground chia seeds, baking powder, and salt in a large mixing bowl until combined. Stir in the yeast mixture, canola oil, and vinegar. Mix well until there are no lumps.

Divide the batter evenly between the ramekins and let rise in a warm space for 20 to 25 minutes until the batter has doubled in size.

Place the ramekins on a large baking sheet and bake for 20 to 25 minutes until golden brown on top. Let the muffins cool completely in the ramekins before turning them out. Slice in half and enjoy. Store in an airtight container for 3 to 4 days or freeze for up to 3 months.

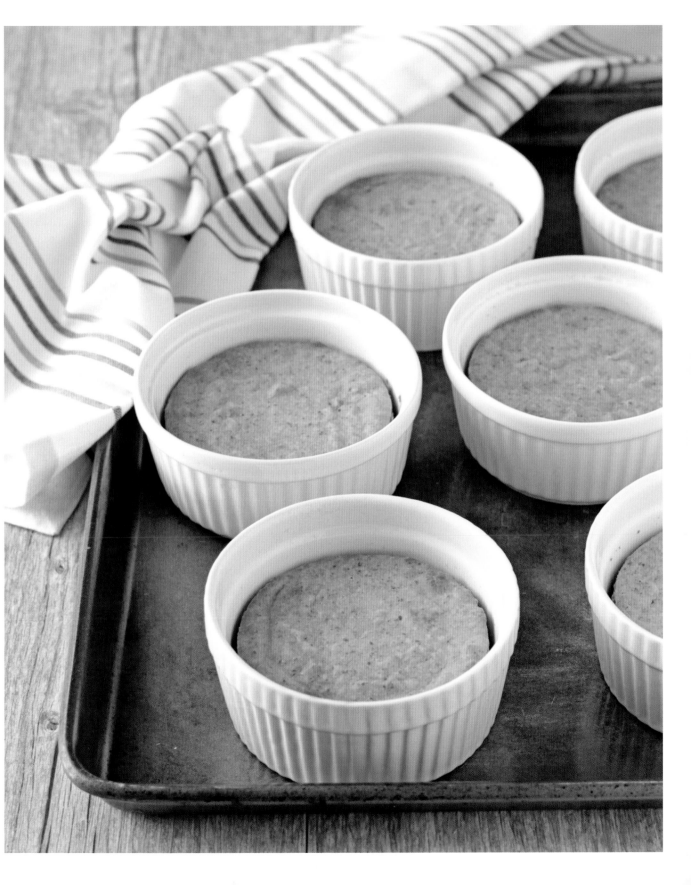

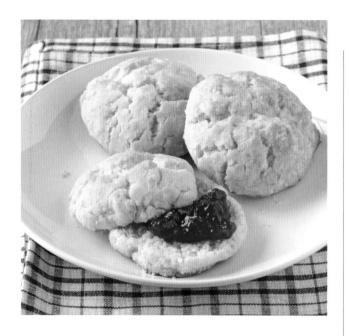

MOM'S BEST BISCUITS

YIELD: 8 BISCUITS

My mom always makes biscuits to accompany stick-to-your-ribs soups and stews, and now that I've figured out how to make them gum-free and low-FODMAP, I do, too. A scaled-down version of these biscuits forms the crust of my Skillet Chicken Pot Pie on page 135—but they're not just sidekicks for savory recipes. These biscuits are also fabulous for breakfast, spread with a little organic strawberry jam.

1½ CUPS (243 G) BASIC FLOUR BLEND (PAGE 38)

½ CUP (60 G) TAPIOCA FLOUR

1 TABLESPOON (13 G) SUGAR

1½ TEASPOONS BAKING POWDER

½ TEASPOON SALT

6 TABLESPOONS (85 G) UNSALTED BUTTER, CUT INTO PIECES AND CHILLED

⅔ CUP (160 ML) LACTOSE-FREE OR NONDAIRY MILK

Preheat the oven to 400°F (200°C, or gas mark 6). Line a baking sheet with parchment paper.

In a large bowl, stir together the Basic Flour Blend, tapioca flour, sugar, baking powder, and salt. Cut in the butter using forks or a pastry blender (or, alternatively, a food processor) until the mixture resembles coarse meal. Add the milk and stir thoroughly until the dough thickens.

Use a ¼-cup (60 ml) scoop or a spring-loaded cupcake scoop to drop biscuit-size portions of the dough onto the prepared baking sheet. Bake for 14 to 16 minutes until the biscuits are lightly browned on top. Let cool for 10 to 15 minutes before slicing. Store for 1 to 2 days in an airtight container or freeze for up to 3 months.

Make it vegan! Replace the butter with vegan margarine, reduce the salt to a teaspoon, and use nondairy milk. (The biscuits won't brown as much if you use unsweetened nondairy milk, but they'll still be done after baking them for 14 to 16 minutes.)

MAPLE CINNAMON CORN BREAD

YIELD: 8 SERVINGS

Sweetened with maple syrup and spiced with a hint of cinnamon, this corn bread is incredibly tender, light, and fluffy since it's made with corn flour instead of corn meal. Bob's Red Mill makes a wonderful gluten-free corn flour, but if you can't find it, try masa harina, which is also gluten-free and is available at most grocery stores. Smear a slice with butter and serve it alongside a bowl of soup, like the Salmon Chowder on page 118.

1 CUP (162 G) BASIC FLOUR BLEND (PAGE 38)

1 CUP (116 G) CORN FLOUR

1 TEASPOON GROUND CINNAMON

½ TEASPOON BAKING POWDER

½ TEASPOON BAKING SODA

½ TEASPOON SALT

2 LARGE EGGS

1 CUP (235 ML) LACTOSE-FREE MILK

½ CUP (120 ML) PURE MAPLE SYRUP

¼ CUP (60 ML) CANOLA OIL OR OTHER NEUTRAL OIL

Preheat the oven to 400°F (200°C, or gas mark 6). Spray a 9-inch (23 cm) round or square baking pan with cooking spray.

In a large bowl, combine the Basic Flour Blend, corn flour, cinnamon, baking powder, baking soda, and salt. In a medium bowl, lightly beat the eggs and stir in the milk, maple syrup, and canola oil. Add the milk mixture to the flour mixture and stir well until there are no lumps.

Pour into the prepared pan and bake for 16 to 18 minutes until a toothpick inserted into the middle of the corn bread comes out clean. Store at room temperature, covered with aluminum foil, for 2 to 3 days.

Make muffins instead! Line a standard-size 12-cup muffin pan with paper liners or coat with cooking spray. Fill each muffin cup two-thirds full with the batter. Bake for 10 to 12 minutes until a toothpick inserted into the center of a muffin comes out clean and the tops are starting to brown.

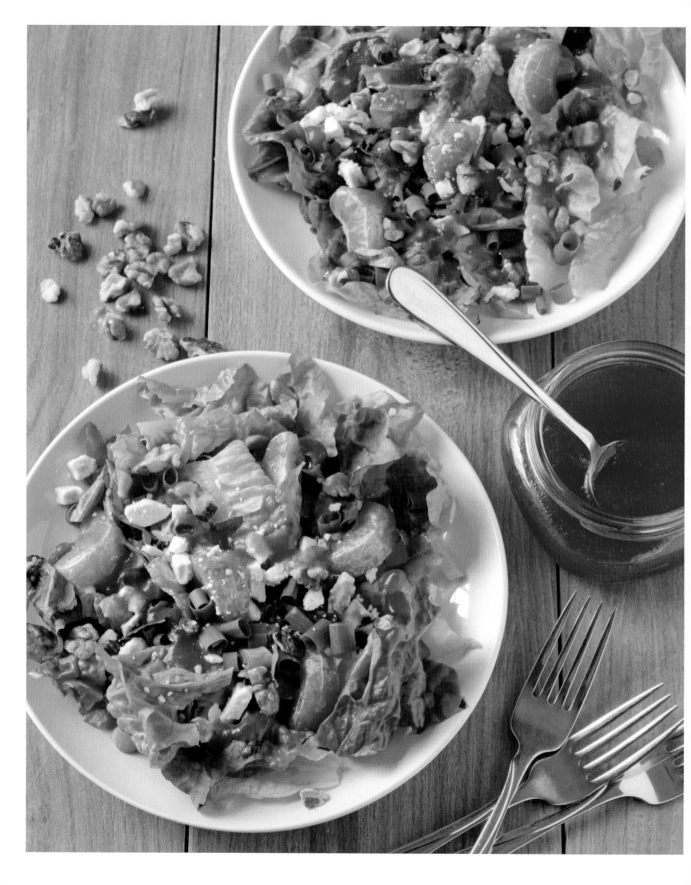

SALADS AND SIDES

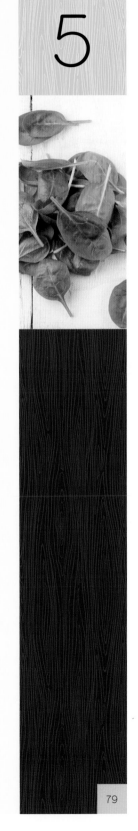

5

Salads and side dishes usually play supporting roles in the dinnertime drama, but if you ask me, they're just as important as the main course. In fact, they're often my favorite part of the meal! So whether you're looking for the perfect dish to complement your favorite meaty main or a salad to throw together for a light lunch, you'll find just what you're after in this chapter. I love salads that feature a vinaigrette dressing, crumbled cheese, and fruit, and there are so many low-FODMAP variations on that theme. Lots of them appear here, like the Balsamic and Blue Spinach Salad on page 81. When it comes to carbs, you'll want to reach for potatoes, rice, and quinoa, which are natural choices when you're on a low-FODMAP diet. Try the Parmesan Garlic Smashed Potatoes on page 88 (you'll never believe they're low-FODMAP!) or German Potato Salad with Goat Cheese and Chives on page 90. And, like rice, quinoa is wonderful when it's served warm in a pilaf (as in Quinoa Pilaf with Carrots and Herbs on page 99), but it's great in salads, too—try the Greek Quinoa Salad on page 85. And if you've got leftovers, don't forget that many of the quinoa and rice dishes included in this chapter can make delicious (and portable!) vegetarian lunches.

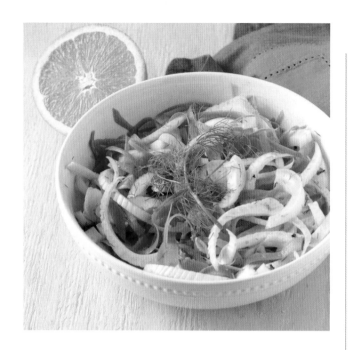

CITRUS FENNEL CARROT SLAW

YIELD: 4 TO 6 SERVINGS

With its refreshing crispness and delicate licorice flavor, fennel is wonderful when it's raw. And since oranges and orange juice are its best friends, it's no surprise that it works so well in a light citrus vinaigrette—mixed with some shredded carrots for an extra pop of color (and a dose of vitamin A). I like to serve this slaw alongside grilled pork chops.

2 TABLESPOONS (28 ML) FRESH ORANGE JUICE

2 TABLESPOONS (28 ML) RICE WINE VINEGAR

1 TABLESPOON (15 ML) OLIVE OIL

1 TABLESPOON (4 G) CHOPPED FENNEL FRONDS

1 TEASPOON SUGAR

1 TEASPOON GRATED ORANGE ZEST

¼ TEASPOON KOSHER SALT

¼ TEASPOON FRESHLY GROUND BLACK PEPPER

1 FENNEL BULB, CUT INTO THIN STRIPS

2 CARROTS, SHREDDED

In a large bowl, whisk together the orange juice, rice wine vinegar, olive oil, fennel fronds, sugar, orange zest, kosher salt, and black pepper. Add the sliced fennel and shredded carrots and toss to coat with the dressing.

Cover and refrigerate for at least 2 hours before serving to let the flavors combine. Store in the refrigerator for up to 2 days.

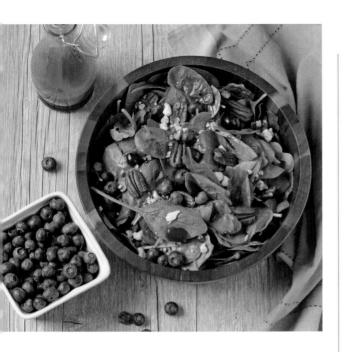

BALSAMIC AND BLUE SPINACH SALAD

YIELD: 4 SERVINGS

Since blue cheese is a hard cheese, it's fairly low in lactose. And that's good news because it adds a huge punch of flavor to this spinach-based salad. So does the balsamic dressing—although it's important to be mindful of the amount of balsamic vinegar you consume in one sitting since it has moderate levels of FODMAPs. Top with grilled chicken breasts for a delightfully healthy lunch.

4 CUPS (120 G) FRESH BABY SPINACH

½ CUP (55 G) PECAN HALVES, TOASTED

½ CUP (75 G) FRESH BLUEBERRIES

¼ CUP (30 G) CRUMBLED BLUE CHEESE

3 TABLESPOONS (45 ML) EXTRA-VIRGIN OLIVE OIL

2 TABLESPOONS (28 ML) BALSAMIC VINEGAR

1 TEASPOON PURE MAPLE SYRUP

½ TEASPOON DIJON MUSTARD

PINCH OF KOSHER SALT

PINCH OF FRESHLY GROUND BLACK PEPPER

In a large bowl, toss together the spinach, pecans, blueberries, and blue cheese.

In a jar or container with a tight-fitting lid, place the olive oil, balsamic vinegar, maple syrup, Dijon mustard, kosher salt, and black pepper. Shake vigorously to combine. Toss the dressing with the salad immediately before serving.

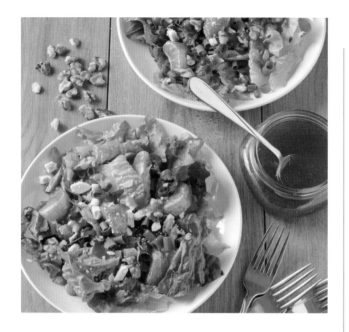

RASPBERRY WALNUT SALAD

YIELD: 4 SERVINGS

This salad is another of my favorites. It boasts a tangy raspberry vinaigrette that's a snap to whisk together (the secret is raspberry jam!), while the mandarin oranges and feta cheese provide complementary sweet-and-salty elements. Just make sure the raspberry jam doesn't contain high-fructose corn syrup; organic brands are usually a good bet. Try it on its own for a light lunch or serve it with grilled fish.

1 PACKAGE (5 OUNCES, OR 140 G) MIXED BABY LETTUCE

½ CUP (75 G) CRUMBLED FETA CHEESE

¼ CUP (30 G) CHOPPED WALNUTS, TOASTED

4 SCALLIONS (GREEN PARTS ONLY), SLICED

2 MANDARIN ORANGES, PEELED AND SECTIONED

2 TABLESPOONS (28 ML) WALNUT OIL

2 TABLESPOONS (28 ML) RED WINE VINEGAR

2 TABLESPOONS (40 G) RASPBERRY JAM (CHECK PRODUCT INGREDIENTS FOR FODMAPS)

2 TABLESPOONS (28 ML) WATER

PINCH OF KOSHER SALT

In a large bowl, toss together the lettuce, feta cheese, walnuts, scallions, and mandarin oranges.

In a jar or container with a tight-fitting lid, place the walnut oil, red wine vinegar, raspberry jam, water, and kosher salt. Shake vigorously to combine. Toss the dressing with the salad immediately before serving.

CAESAR SALAD

YIELD: 4 SERVINGS

There's nothing better than a good Caesar salad—and this one is pretty darn good, if I do say so myself! My aunt makes the best Caesar dressing ever, and my dressing is an adaptation of her recipe. Use Homemade Garlic Oil (page 42) to add a hint of garlic flavor and don't skip the anchovy paste: It adds umami, or savoriness, and it goes so well with Parmesan cheese. Be aware that anchovy paste has not been tested for FODMAPs, so be sure to check the product label for FODMAP ingredients. Use your favorite gluten-free, low-FODMAP bread, either store-bought or homemade, to make the croutons.

2 SLICES OF GLUTEN-FREE SANDWICH, BREAD CUT INTO 1-INCH (2.5 CM) SQUARES

3 TABLESPOONS (45 ML) HOMEMADE GARLIC OIL (PAGE 42) MADE WITH OLIVE OIL, DIVIDED

½ TEASPOON ITALIAN HERB SEASONING (PAGE 40)

2 PINCHES OF KOSHER SALT

2 TABLESPOONS (28 G) LIGHT MAYONNAISE

4 TEASPOONS (20 ML) FRESH LEMON JUICE

1 TEASPOON DIJON MUSTARD

½ TEASPOON ANCHOVY PASTE (CHECK PRODUCT INGREDIENTS FOR FODMAPS)

¼ TEASPOON FRESHLY GROUND BLACK PEPPER

PINCH OF KOSHER SALT

6 CUPS (282 G) TORN ROMAINE HEARTS

¼ CUP (25 G) GRATED PARMESAN CHEESE

Preheat the oven to 300°F (150°C, or gas mark 2). To make the croutons, place the bread pieces in a shallow baking dish. Toss with 1 tablespoon (15 ml) (or less, if desired) of the garlic oil, the Italian herb seasoning, and a pinch of kosher salt. Bake for 20 minutes, stirring several times, until the bread is lightly toasted. Let cool.

In a large bowl, whisk together the remaining 2 tablespoons (28 ml) garlic oil, mayonnaise, lemon juice, Dijon mustard, anchovy paste, black pepper, and the remaining pinch of kosher salt. Add the Romaine lettuce, Parmesan cheese, and croutons to the bowl with the dressing and toss. Serve immediately.

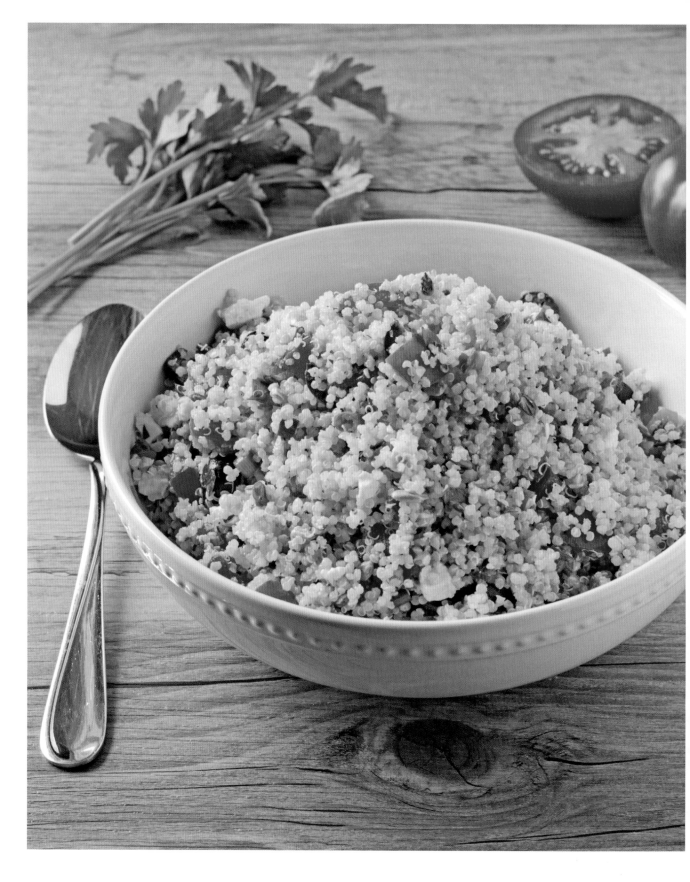

GREEK QUINOA SALAD

YIELD: 6 SERVINGS

This gluten-free take on a Greek pasta salad is laden with strong flavors—think tomato, olives, feta, and fresh parsley—and it boasts an added layer of texture from roasted sunflower seeds. It's a big hit at potlucks and barbecues: I often bring it along to share so that I know I'll have a low-FODMAP choice, and everyone else really enjoys it, too.

1 CUP (173 G) QUINOA, RINSED

1½ CUPS (355 ML) WATER

¾ TEASPOON KOSHER SALT, DIVIDED

1 CUP (180 G) CHOPPED TOMATOES

1 CAN (2.25 OUNCES, OR 62 G) SLICED BLACK OLIVES, DRAINED

½ CUP (75 G) CRUMBLED FETA CHEESE

¼ CUP (36 G) ROASTED UNSALTED SUNFLOWER SEEDS

4 SCALLIONS (GREEN PARTS ONLY), SLICED

¼ CUP (15 G) CHOPPED FRESH ITALIAN PARSLEY

¼ CUP (60 ML) FRESH LEMON JUICE

2 TABLESPOONS (28 ML) EXTRA-VIRGIN OLIVE OIL

1 TEASPOON DIJON MUSTARD

¼ TEASPOON FRESHLY GROUND BLACK PEPPER

In a medium saucepan, combine the quinoa, water, and ½ teaspoon of the kosher salt. Bring to a boil over high heat. Reduce the heat to low, cover, and simmer for 15 to 20 minutes until most of the water is absorbed. Keeping the pan covered, remove it from the heat and let it steam for 5 to 10 minutes. Spread the quinoa on a baking sheet and let cool, about 30 minutes.

Transfer the cooled quinoa to a large bowl. Add the tomatoes, black olives, feta cheese, sunflower seeds, scallions, and parsley. Toss to combine.

In a small bowl, whisk together the lemon juice, olive oil, Dijon mustard, the remaining ¼ teaspoon kosher salt, and the black pepper.

Pour the lemon dressing over the quinoa salad and toss. Serve immediately or store in the refrigerator for up to 2 days.

CHICKEN SALAD WITH PECANS AND GRAPES

YIELD: 4 TO 6 SERVINGS

This easy-to-make chicken salad is perfect for workday lunches—even if you're eating at your desk. Use it to top rice cakes or rice crackers or serve it with cooked, cooled quinoa, and you've got a quick, filling, healthy lunch in an instant. It's a great way to use up leftover roasted chicken, but you can also use poached chicken breasts or the meat of a rotisserie chicken instead.

2 CUPS (280 G) CHOPPED COOKED CHICKEN

2 SCALLIONS (GREEN PARTS ONLY), SLICED

¾ CUP (113 G) RED GRAPES, HALVED

½ OF A STALK OF CELERY, FINELY DICED

¼ CUP (28 G) CHOPPED TOASTED PECAN HALVES

1 TABLESPOON (4 G) CHOPPED FRESH ITALIAN PARSLEY

⅓ CUP (75 G) LIGHT MAYONNAISE

¼ TEASPOON KOSHER SALT

¼ TEASPOON FRESHLY GROUND BLACK PEPPER

Combine the chicken, scallions, grapes, celery, pecans, and parsley in a medium bowl. Fold in the mayonnaise and season with the kosher salt and black pepper. Serve immediately or store in the refrigerator for up to 2 days.

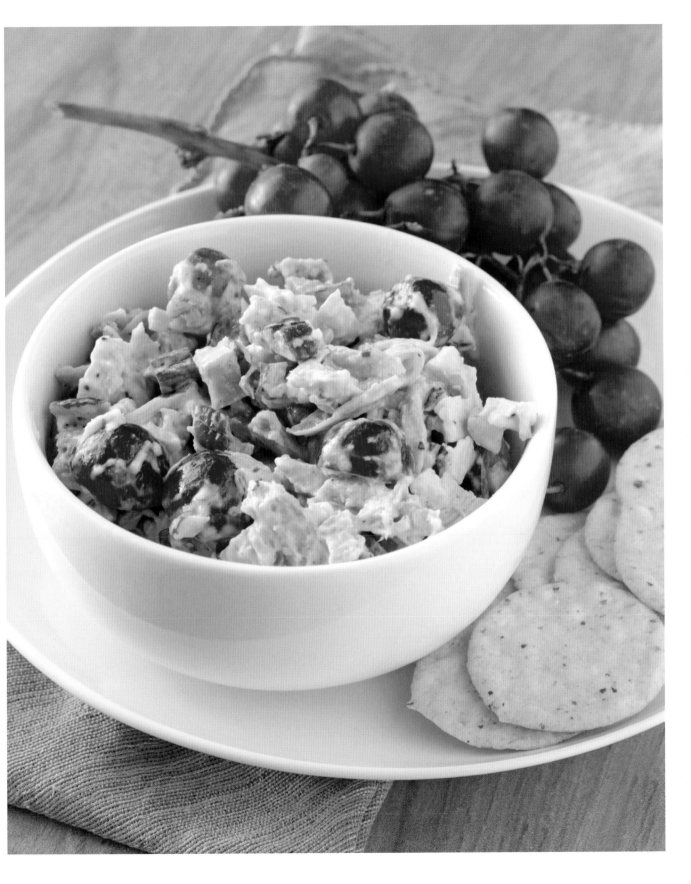

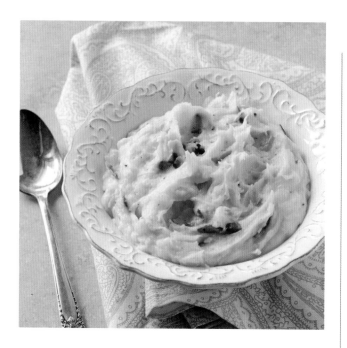

PARMESAN GARLIC SMASHED POTATOES

YIELD: 4 SERVINGS

Wait, *garlic* smashed potatoes? That's right. Don't worry: They're flavored with garlic oil instead of whole garlic, making them a safe low-FODMAP choice. These smashed potatoes are perfect as a side dish or in Turkey Shepherd's Pie (page 137). Leave the thin, tender skins of the red potatoes intact to give this comforting side dish an extra helping of fiber.

1½ POUNDS (680 G) RED POTATOES (ABOUT 8 SMALL), QUARTERED, SKIN ON

1½ TEASPOONS KOSHER SALT, DIVIDED

2 TABLESPOONS (28 ML) HOMEMADE GARLIC OIL (PAGE 42)

2 TABLESPOONS (28 G) UNSALTED BUTTER OR MARGARINE

½ CUP (40 G) SHREDDED PARMESAN CHEESE

¼ TEASPOON FRESHLY GROUND BLACK PEPPER

½ CUP (120 ML) LACTOSE-FREE OR NONDAIRY MILK

Place the potatoes in a large pot or Dutch oven. Add enough water to cover the potatoes. Stir in 1 teaspoon of the kosher salt. Bring to a boil, then reduce the heat, cover, and simmer for 25 to 30 minutes until they pierce easily when you insert a paring knife.

Meanwhile, pour the garlic oil into the bowl of a stand mixer. Add the butter, Parmesan cheese, the remaining ½ teaspoon kosher salt, and the black pepper.

Remove the potatoes from the heat and drain. Add them to the mixer bowl with the other ingredients and mix on medium speed until smooth. Slowly add the milk until the desired consistency is achieved. Serve hot.

ROSEMARY ROASTED RED POTATOES

YIELD: 4 SERVINGS

This is my all-time favorite potato recipe, and I end up making it at least once a week. It's simplicity itself and it's really healthy—and plus, the potatoes turn out gloriously golden and crispy. To sneak extra veggies into your meal, you can add a few cups (120 g) of raw baby spinach to the potatoes before briefly popping them back into the oven: It'll cook in no time, and, more important, it's loaded with essential vitamins and minerals.

1½ POUNDS (680 G) RED POTATOES, CUT INTO WEDGES

2 TABLESPOONS (28 ML) OLIVE OIL

2 SPRIGS FRESH ROSEMARY, MINCED (OR 1 TEASPOON DRIED, CRUSHED)

½ TEASPOON KOSHER SALT

½ TEASPOON FRESHLY GROUND BLACK PEPPER

4 CUPS (120 G) FRESH BABY SPINACH (OPTIONAL)

Preheat the oven to 425°F (220°C, or gas mark 7). Lightly grease a baking sheet with cooking spray. (For easier cleanup, line the sheet with aluminum foil before spraying.)

In a large bowl, toss the potatoes with the olive oil, rosemary, kosher salt, and black pepper. Spread the potatoes on the baking sheet and bake for 25 to 30 minutes, stirring occasionally, until golden brown.

Remove the potatoes from the oven and stir in the spinach (if desired). Return to the oven for 1 to 2 minutes more until the spinach is wilted. Serve hot.

GERMAN POTATO SALAD WITH GOAT CHEESE AND CHIVES

YIELD: 4 SERVINGS

Doused in a Dijon vinaigrette and served warm, this potato salad is even more comforting than the traditional picnic-table version that's loaded with mayo. (Then again, maybe that's just my German heritage talking!) Minced chives give it a fresh, oniony flavor, and the goat cheese lends it a tangy creaminess. Like my Greek Quinoa Salad on page 85, it's an ideal dish for sharing at summertime barbecues.

1½ POUNDS (680 G) RED POTATOES, CUT INTO ¾-INCH (2 CM) CUBES

1¼ TEASPOONS KOSHER SALT, DIVIDED

4 SLICES OF BACON, CUT INTO ½-INCH (1.3 CM) STRIPS

¼ CUP (60 ML) RICE WINE VINEGAR

1 TABLESPOON (15 G) DIJON MUSTARD

½ TEASPOON FRESHLY GROUND BLACK PEPPER

½ CUP (75 G) CRUMBLED GOAT CHEESE

2 TABLESPOONS (6 G) MINCED FRESH CHIVES

Place the potatoes in a large saucepan and cover with about an inch (2.5 cm) of water. Add 1 teaspoon of the kosher salt. Bring to a boil over high heat. Reduce the heat to medium. Simmer the potatoes, uncovered, for about 8 minutes (the potatoes will still be a little underdone).

While the potatoes are cooking, fry the bacon in a large skillet over medium heat until crispy. Transfer the bacon to a paper towel and drain the bacon grease from the pan (but don't wipe it clean). Return the bacon to the skillet and add the rice wine vinegar, Dijon mustard, the remaining ¼ teaspoon kosher salt, and black pepper to the skillet. Bring to a simmer over medium heat.

Stir in the potatoes and cook until the liquid is mostly absorbed, about 5 minutes. Gently toss in the goat cheese and minced fresh chives. Serve warm.

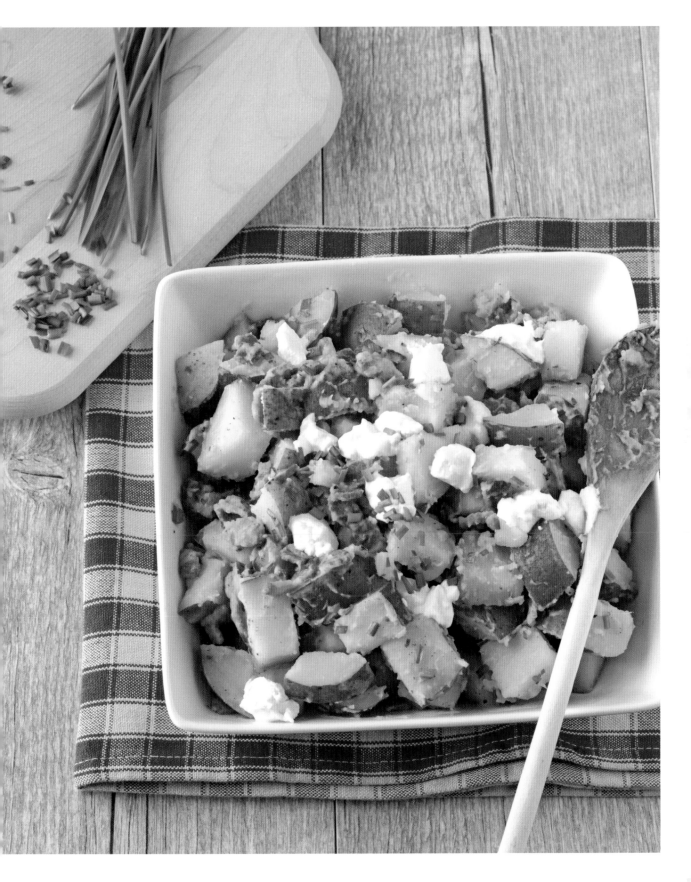

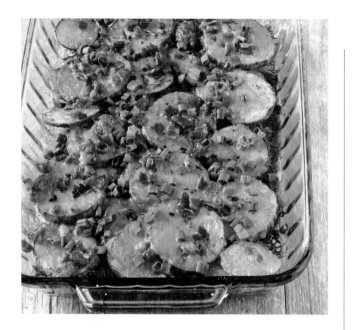

LOADED BAKED POTATO COINS

YIELD: 4 SERVINGS

You know those deep-fried potato skins stuffed with bacon, cheese, and sour cream? They may be chain-restaurant staples, but boy, are they addictive! These baked potato "coins" are a healthier, low-FODMAP take on those not-so-good-for-you snacks. And they're much easier to make. If you're a fan of twice-baked potatoes—or anything involving crisp potatoes and cheese, for that matter—you're sure to love them as much as I do.

2 LARGE RUSSET POTATOES (ABOUT 1½ POUNDS, OR 680 G), CUT INTO ¼-INCH (6 MM) SLICES

2 TABLESPOONS (28 G) UNSALTED BUTTER, MELTED

½ TEASPOON KOSHER SALT

¼ TEASPOON FRESHLY GROUND BLACK PEPPER

4 SLICES OF BACON, COOKED UNTIL CRISP, THEN DRAINED AND CRUMBLED

1 CUP (120 G) SHREDDED CHEDDAR CHEESE

2 SCALLIONS (GREEN PARTS ONLY), SLICED

Preheat the oven to 425°F (220°C, or gas mark 7). Spray a 9 x 13-inch (23 x 33 cm) baking pan with cooking spray.

Arrange the potatoes in the bottom of the prepared pan. Drizzle with the melted butter and sprinkle with the kosher salt and black pepper. Bake for 20 to 25 minutes, stirring once, until the potatoes are easily pierced with a knife.

Remove the potato coins from the oven. Sprinkle them with the bacon and shredded cheddar cheese and bake for 5 minutes more until the cheese is melted. Sprinkle with the sliced scallions and serve.

SAUTÉED SWISS CHARD

YIELD: 4 SERVINGS

I first tried Swiss chard just a couple of years ago, and these days, I'm making up for lost time! And it turns out that you can actually eat the whole leaf, including the stems (the stems take longer to cook, which is why I add them to the skillet first). Swiss chard is really delicious when it's simply sautéed, then topped with lemon juice and Parmesan cheese. It goes well with almost anything—including roasted chicken or grilled steak or salmon.

4 CUPS (144 G) SLICED SWISS CHARD, STEMS AND LEAVES SEPARATED

1 TABLESPOON (15 ML) OLIVE OIL

1 CLOVE OF GARLIC, PEELED AND SMASHED, BUT KEPT WHOLE

2 TEASPOONS FRESH LEMON JUICE

⅛ TEASPOON KOSHER SALT

⅛ TEASPOON FRESHLY GROUND BLACK PEPPER

¼ CUP (25 G) GRATED PARMESAN CHEESE

Cut the chard leaves crosswise into 1-inch (2.5 cm) strips. Slice the stems.

Heat the olive oil in a large skillet over medium heat. Add the garlic and sauté until starting to brown. Remove the garlic from the skillet and discard. Add the chard stems and sauté for about 5 minutes. Add the chard leaves and sauté for another 3 to 4 minutes. Stir in the lemon juice, kosher salt, and black pepper. Sprinkle with the Parmesan cheese just before serving.

ROASTED GREEN BEANS AND PROSCIUTTO

YIELD: 4 SERVINGS

Green beans are low in FODMAPs, but it's important to be mindful of the serving size. Fortunately, this recipe is carefully calibrated to give you four low-FODMAP servings. If you are as big a fan of the humble green bean as I am, you will love this recipe. Roasting them enhances both their flavor and their texture, so you're sure to love this twist on the classic green-beans-and-bacon combo.

½ POUND (225 G) FRESH GREEN BEANS, TRIMMED

2 SLICES OF PROSCIUTTO, CUT INTO ½-INCH (1.3 CM) STRIPS

⅛ TEASPOON KOSHER SALT

⅛ TEASPOON FRESHLY GROUND BLACK PEPPER

Preheat the oven to 400°F (200°C, or gas mark 6). Line a large rimmed baking sheet with aluminum foil. Lightly coat with cooking spray. Lay the green beans out on the sheet in a single layer. Lightly spritz the beans with cooking spray as well. Sprinkle them with the prosciutto, kosher salt, and black pepper.

Bake for 10 minutes and then stir. Bake for another 5 to 10 minutes until the green beans are browned and the prosciutto is crispy. Serve immediately.

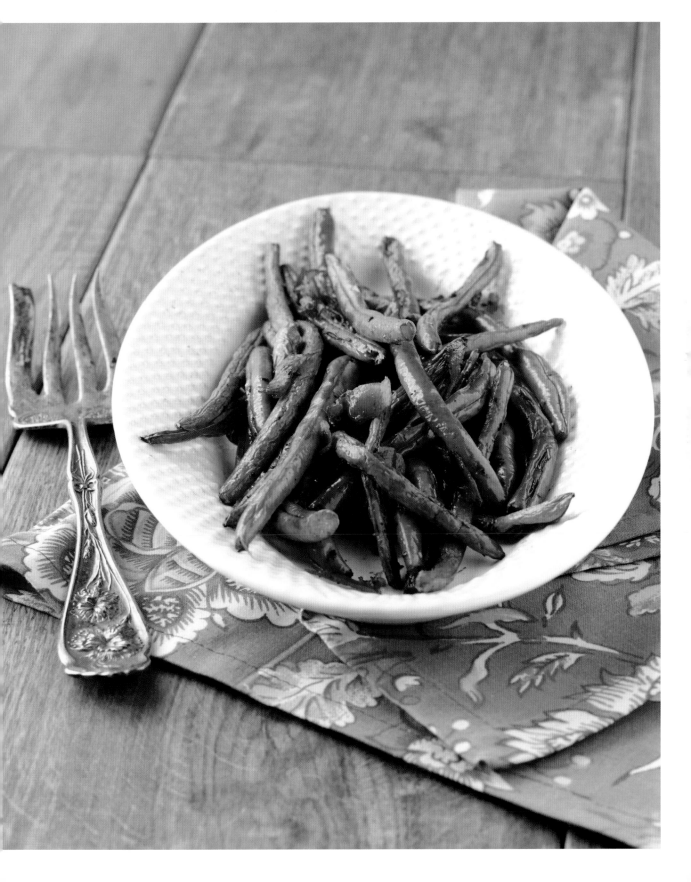

SPINACH QUINOA TABBOULEH

YIELD: 4 SERVINGS

Tabbouleh, a vegetarian Middle Eastern dish, is usually made with bulgur or couscous, both of which are made from wheat. But this low-FODMAP version calls for gluten-free quinoa, since it's a small grain with a similar texture to couscous. Because it's chock-full of spinach, fresh mint, tomatoes, and cucumbers, it's really refreshing, and it can work either as a side dish or a vegan main course. This recipe was inspired by *Real Simple* magazine.

1 CUP (173 G) QUINOA, RINSED

1½ CUPS (355 ML) WATER

¾ TEASPOON KOSHER SALT

¼ CUP (60 ML) EXTRA-VIRGIN OLIVE OIL

1 CLOVE OF GARLIC, PEELED AND SMASHED, BUT KEPT WHOLE

3 TABLESPOONS (45 ML) FRESH LEMON JUICE

¼ TEASPOON FRESHLY GROUND BLACK PEPPER

4 CUPS (120 G) FRESH BABY SPINACH

½ CUP (48 G) FRESH MINT LEAVES

1 LARGE TOMATO, CHOPPED (ABOUT 1 CUP, OR 180 G)

1 CUP (135 G) CHOPPED CUCUMBER

4 SCALLIONS (GREEN PARTS ONLY), SLICED

In a large saucepan, bring the quinoa, water, and ½ teaspoon of the kosher salt to a boil. Reduce the heat to low, cover, and simmer for 15 to 20 minutes until most of the water is absorbed. Keeping the pan covered, remove it from the heat and let it steam for 5 to 10 minutes.

Meanwhile, heat the olive oil in a small skillet over medium heat. Add the garlic clove and sauté for 1½ to 2 minutes. Remove the garlic from the oil (and discard) before it starts to brown. Remove the skillet from the heat and let cool.

In a small bowl, whisk together the cooled garlic oil, lemon juice, remaining ¼ teaspoon kosher salt, and the black pepper.

Place the spinach and mint leaves in a food processor and pulse until finely chopped. Toss the cooked quinoa, garlic oil mixture, chopped spinach and mint, tomato, cucumber, and scallions together in a bowl. Serve at room temperature or chilled.

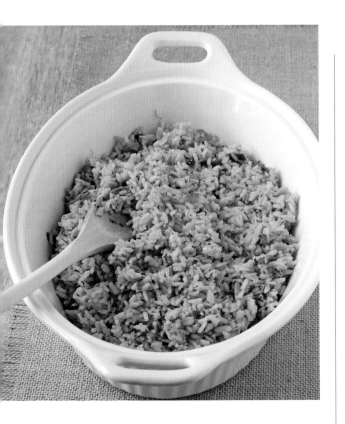

BAKED BROWN RICE WITH PARMESAN AND HERBS

YIELD: 6 SERVINGS

Several years ago, I learned that the best way to prepare brown rice is by baking it. Other methods, like boiling, usually left me with undercooked rice with a pasty texture—but baking the rice makes it perfectly tender and fluffy every time. (If you can find it, use brown basmati rice—it lends the dish a nuttier flavor—but if not, regular long-grain brown rice works fine, too.) Dress it up with herbs, Parmesan cheese, and pine nuts and serve with grilled chicken or fish.

1½ CUPS (294 G) BROWN BASMATI RICE

2 TEASPOONS DRIED BASIL

1 TEASPOON DRIED THYME

1 TEASPOON KOSHER SALT

½ TEASPOON FRESHLY GROUND BLACK PEPPER

1 TABLESPOON (15 ML) OLIVE OIL

1 CLOVE OF GARLIC, PEELED AND SMASHED, BUT KEPT WHOLE

1⅓ CUPS (315 ML) WATER

1 CUP (235 ML) CHICKEN STOCK OR CHICKEN BROTH (PAGE 109 OR 110)

⅓ CUP (45 G) PINE NUTS, TOASTED

¼ CUP (15 G) CHOPPED FRESH ITALIAN PARSLEY

¼ CUP (25 G) SLICED SCALLIONS (GREEN PARTS ONLY)

¼ CUP (25 G) GRATED PARMESAN CHEESE

Preheat the oven to 375°F (190°C, or gas mark 5). Combine the brown rice, basil, thyme, kosher salt, and black pepper in a 2½-quart (2.4 L) casserole dish.

Heat the olive oil in a large saucepan over medium heat. Add the garlic and cook until it starts to brown. Remove and discard the garlic. Add the water and chicken stock or broth to the pan, increase the heat to high, and bring to a boil. Remove from the heat and carefully pour the liquid into the casserole dish with the rice and seasonings.

Cover the dish and bake for 1 hour or until the liquid is absorbed and the rice is tender. Fluff the rice and then stir in the pine nuts, chopped fresh parsley, sliced scallions, and Parmesan cheese. Serve immediately.

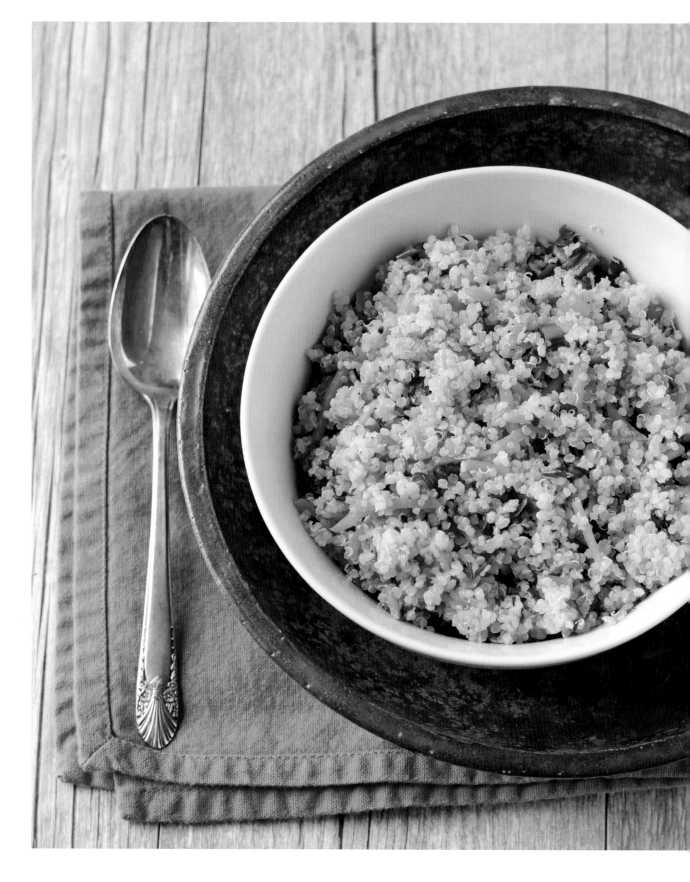

QUINOA PILAF WITH CARROTS AND HERBS

YIELD: 4 SERVINGS

This simple quinoa pilaf is a lovely partner for countless main courses, and it can act as a vegan main course in its own right, too: Just use vegetable broth and add some sautéed tempeh. Toasting the quinoa and cooking it in broth or stock lends it a fuller, richer flavor, so don't be tempted to skip that step! Finish the pilaf with a handful of fresh herbs, if you like. I'm partial to thyme, but feel free to toss in your favorites along with the parsley just before serving.

1 TABLESPOON (15 ML) OLIVE OIL

1 CLOVE OF GARLIC, PEELED AND SMASHED, BUT KEPT WHOLE

1 CUP (173 G) QUINOA, RINSED

1½ CUPS (355 ML) CHICKEN BROTH, CHICKEN STOCK, OR VEGETABLE BROTH (PAGE 110, 109, OR 112)

½ CUP (55 G) SHREDDED CARROTS

½ TEASPOON DRIED THYME

½ TEASPOON KOSHER SALT

¼ TEASPOON FRESHLY GROUND BLACK PEPPER

4 SCALLIONS (GREEN PARTS ONLY), SLICED

¼ CUP (15 G) CHOPPED FRESH ITALIAN PARSLEY

Heat the olive oil in a large saucepan over medium heat. Add the garlic and cook until softened, about 1 to 2 minutes. Remove and discard the garlic. Add the quinoa to the oil and sauté until lightly browned, about 5 minutes.

Add the broth or stock, shredded carrots, thyme, kosher salt, and black pepper. Bring the mixture to a boil and then reduce the heat to low. Cover and simmer for 15 to 20 minutes until most of the water is absorbed. Keeping the pan covered, remove it from the heat and let it steam for 5 to 10 minutes. Stir in the sliced scallions and chopped fresh parsley and serve.

CILANTRO LIME RICE

YIELD: 4 SERVINGS

If you're making the Beef Tacos on page 148 or the Pork Carnitas on page 158, you've got to make a batch of this fluffy, flavorful rice to serve alongside it: It's one of my all-time favorites. Are you not a fan of cilantro? (Some folks are turned off by a perceived "soapy" taste.) That's no problem: Parsley works just as well in its place.

1 TABLESPOON (15 ML) OLIVE OIL

1 CLOVE OF GARLIC, PEELED

1 CUP (192 G) WHITE BASMATI RICE
(OR LONG-GRAIN WHITE RICE)

1½ CUPS (355 ML) WATER

1 TEASPOON KOSHER SALT

¼ CUP (4 G) CHOPPED FRESH CILANTRO

3 SCALLIONS (GREEN PARTS ONLY), SLICED

1 TABLESPOON (15 ML) FRESH LIME JUICE

¼ TEASPOON GRATED LIME ZEST

½ TEASPOON GROUND CUMIN

¼ TEASPOON FRESHLY GROUND BLACK PEPPER

Heat the olive oil in a large saucepan over medium heat. Add the garlic and cook until it starts to brown. Remove and discard the garlic. Add the rice to the oil in the saucepan and sauté until the rice is very lightly toasted, about 3 to 5 minutes. Add the water and kosher salt. Bring to a boil, reduce the heat to low, and cover. Simmer for 15 to 20 minutes until the water is mostly absorbed. Keeping the pan covered, remove it from the heat and let sit for 10 to 15 minutes to steam.

Stir in the chopped fresh cilantro, sliced scallions, lime juice, lime zest, cumin, and black pepper. Serve hot.

SUMMER GARDEN SLOW COOKER RISOTTO

YIELD: 6 SERVINGS

Slow cookers are usually associated with wintertime soups and casseroles, but there's no need to shove yours into the back of the pantry when the weather warms up! They're especially handy in summer since they won't heat up your kitchen as much as an oven or stove will. And they make such easy work of labor-intensive risotto. This dish incorporates lots of your summer garden vegetables and herbs—like zucchini, tomatoes, and basil—and the best part is, there's no stirring involved! This recipe was inspired by a similar one on allrecipes.com.

1¼ CUPS (240 G) ARBORIO RICE

¼ CUP (60 ML) HOMEMADE GARLIC OIL (PAGE 42)

3¾ CUPS (880 ML) CHICKEN BROTH, CHICKEN STOCK, OR VEGETABLE BROTH (PAGE 110, 109, OR 112)

¼ CUP (60 ML) DRY WHITE WINE (OR BROTH OR STOCK)

1½ TEASPOONS KOSHER SALT

¼ TEASPOON FRESHLY GROUND BLACK PEPPER

2 CUPS (240 G) CHOPPED ZUCCHINI

4 SCALLIONS (GREEN PARTS ONLY), THINLY SLICED

¼ CUP (10 G) CHOPPED FRESH BASIL OR 2 TEASPOONS DRIED

1 CUP (180 G) CHOPPED TOMATOES

½ CUP (50 G) GRATED PARMESAN CHEESE, PLUS MORE FOR SERVING (OPTIONAL)

Place the arborio rice and garlic oil in a large slow cooker and stir to coat the rice with the garlic oil. Stir in the broth, white wine (or additional broth or stock), kosher salt, and black pepper. Finally, stir in the zucchini, scallions, and basil. Cover and cook on high for about 2 hours or until most of the liquid is absorbed.

Stir in the tomatoes and Parmesan cheese and continue to cook on high until heated through, about 5 to 10 minutes. Serve with more Parmesan cheese sprinkled on top, if you like.

GREEK BLISTERED-TOMATO PASTA

YIELD: 4 SERVINGS

When I saw a photo of a recipe just like this one in a grocery store ad—no recipe included—I knew I had to re-create it myself. And I did! This low-FODMAP Greek-inspired pasta features cherry tomatoes that are sautéed until they blister, and they're delicious when they pop in your mouth. It's especially good when it's served alongside a simple baked tilapia: Sprinkle tilapia fillets with lemon juice, kosher salt, black pepper, and paprika and bake at 425°F (220°C, or gas mark 7) for about 10 minutes while you prepare the pasta.

8 OUNCES (225 G) GLUTEN-FREE RICE SPAGHETTI

2 TABLESPOONS (28 ML) OLIVE OIL

1 CLOVE OF GARLIC, PEELED AND SMASHED, BUT KEPT WHOLE

1 CUP (150 G) CHERRY TOMATOES

4 CUPS (120 G) FRESH BABY SPINACH

½ CUP (85 G) KALAMATA OLIVES, DRAINED

1 TEASPOON ANCHOVY PASTE (CHECK PRODUCT INGREDIENTS FOR FODMAPS)

½ TEASPOON DRIED OREGANO

½ TEASPOON KOSHER SALT

¼ TEASPOON FRESHLY GROUND BLACK PEPPER

½ CUP (75 G) CRUMBLED FETA CHEESE

Bring a large pot of lightly salted water to a boil. Add the spaghetti and cook according to the package directions. Set aside ¼ cup (60 ml) of the cooking liquid. Drain the spaghetti and rinse under cold running water.

Heat the olive oil in a large skillet over medium heat. Add the garlic and cook until it starts to brown. Remove the garlic from the pan and discard. Add the cherry tomatoes and sauté until they start to blister or pop, about 1½ to 2 minutes. Reduce the heat to low and stir in the spinach, Kalmata olives, and anchovy paste. Continue sautéing until the spinach is wilted, about 3 to 4 minutes. Season with the oregano, kosher salt, and black pepper.

Toss the drained spaghetti into the tomato mixture using a pair of tongs, adding the reserved pasta liquid to keep the pasta from sticking. Cook just until heated through. Stir in the feta cheese and serve immediately.

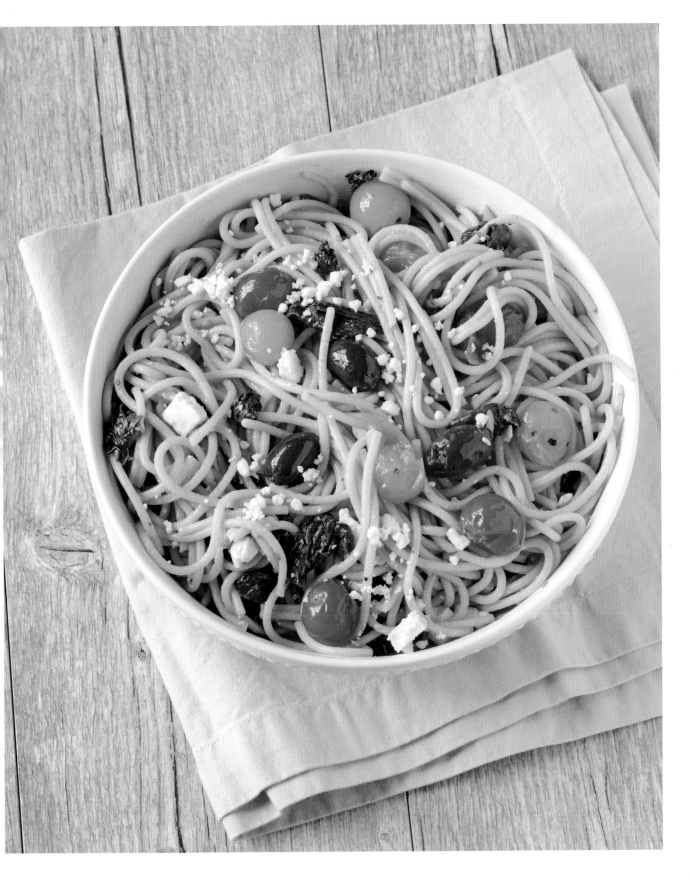

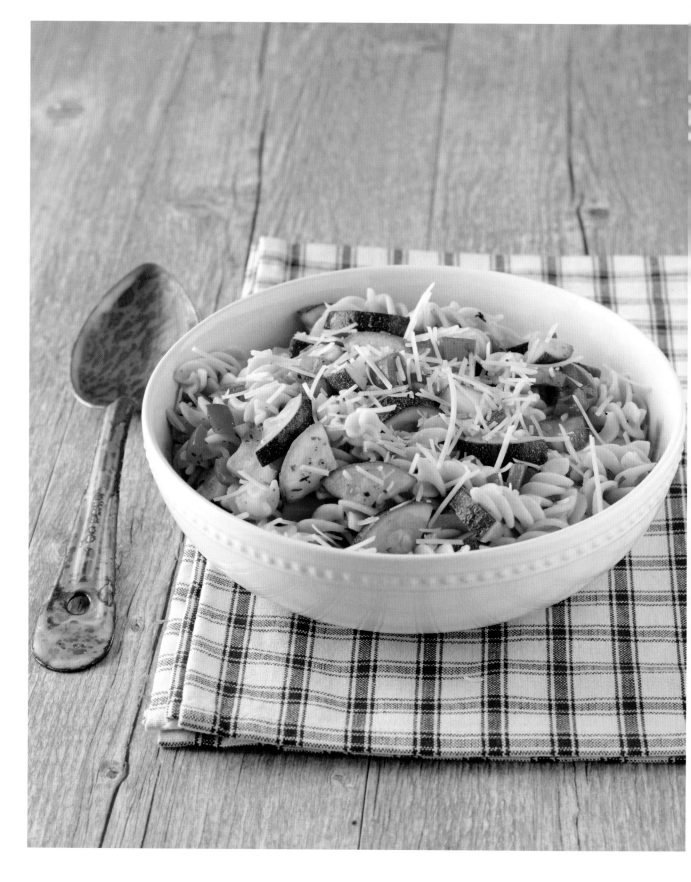

SAUTÉED ZUCCHINI PASTA

YIELD: 4 SERVINGS

With just a handful of ingredients, this simple pasta dish is what's for dinner when zucchini is in season and plentiful. You can pair it with just about anything (or enjoy it on its own), but it's a great supporting act for grilled chicken or baked fish. Or, toss some sautéed shrimp on top.

2 CUPS (224 G) GLUTEN-FREE ROTINI OR FUSILLI PASTA

1 TABLESPOON (15 ML) OLIVE OIL

1 CLOVE OF GARLIC, PEELED AND SMASHED, BUT KEPT WHOLE

1 LARGE ZUCCHINI, QUARTERED LENGTHWISE AND SLICED

½ OF A RED BELL PEPPER, CHOPPED

1 TEASPOON ITALIAN HERB SEASONING (PAGE 40)

½ TEASPOON KOSHER SALT

¼ TEASPOON FRESHLY GROUND BLACK PEPPER

¼ CUP (25 G) GRATED PARMESAN CHEESE

Bring a large pot of lightly salted water to a boil. Cook the pasta according to the package directions. Drain and rinse under cold running water.

Heat the olive oil in a large skillet over medium heat. Add the garlic and sauté until browned. Remove and discard the garlic. Add the zucchini and red bell pepper and sauté until lightly browned and tender, about 8 to 10 minutes. Season with the Italian herb seasoning, kosher salt, and black pepper. Add the pasta to the skillet and toss to combine. Cook until the pasta is just heated through. Serve sprinkled with the Parmesan cheese.

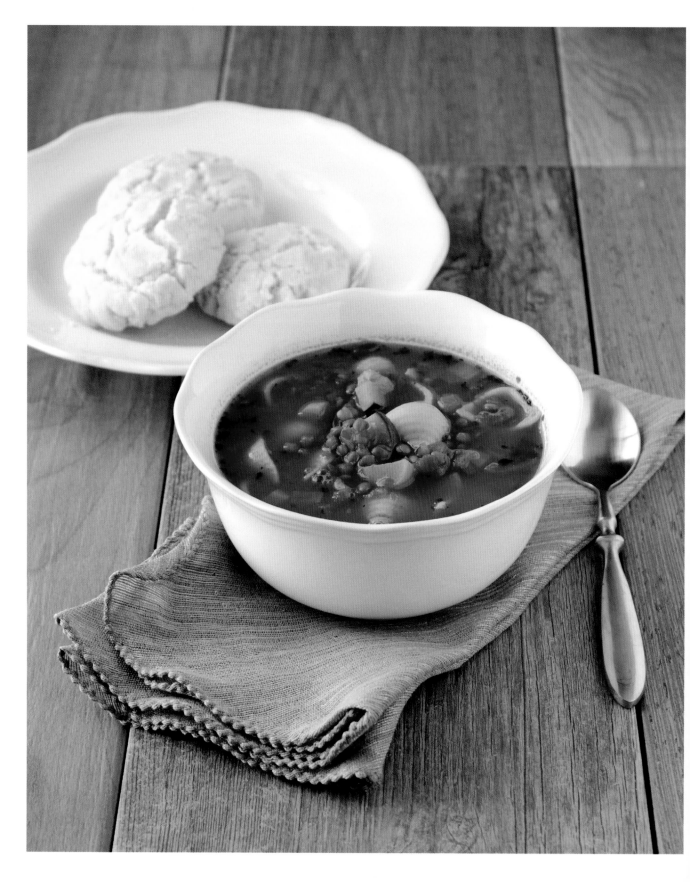

SOUPS AND STEWS

6

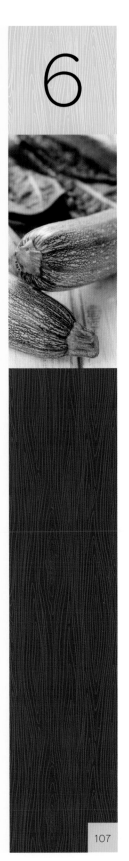

Thanks to the frigid winter weather, growing up in the Midwest taught me to relish warm, comforting soups and stews—the kind that warm you right down to the bones when the thermometer drops below freezing. And the starting point for any soup is a batch of broth or stock. If you're eating low-FODMAP, it's essential that you make your own broths and stocks since there are almost no low-FODMAP packaged broths on the market (most contain onion). Luckily, broths and stocks are really easy to whip up, and I'll show you how to make three different kinds: chicken, beef, and vegetable. Then, I'll teach you how to transform them into flavorful, nourishing soups and hearty stews, like the Creamy Ham and Potato Soup on page 114, the Italian Wedding Soup on page 117, and the Curried Lamb Stew on page 123. Plus, it's a good idea to have homemade broths and stocks in reserve when you're making other recipes in this book since they add extra flavor to casseroles and rice- and quinoa-based side dishes. Freeze broths and stocks in individual portions so that you'll always have just the right amount on hand.

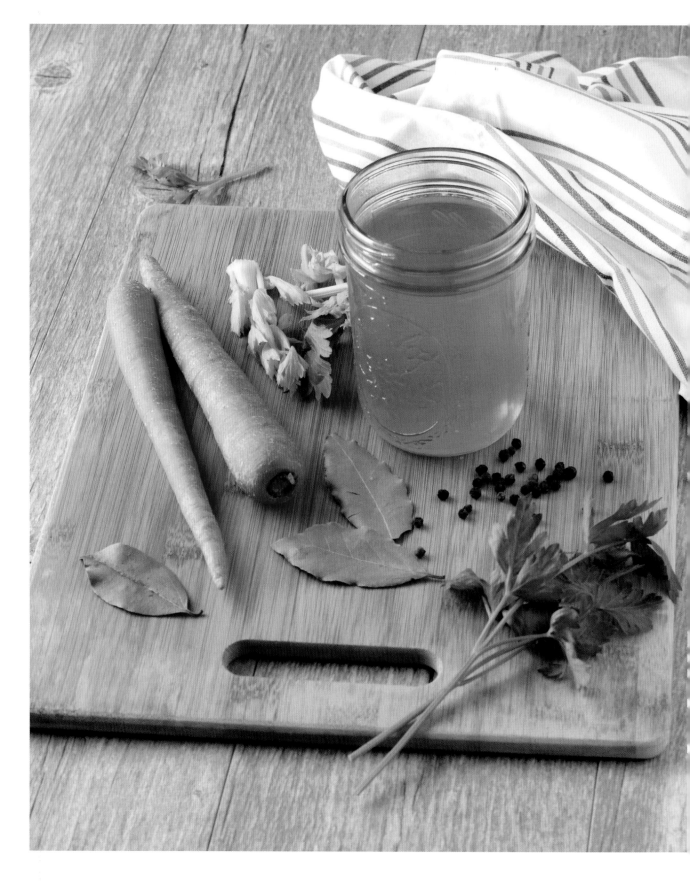

CHICKEN STOCK (BONE BROTH)

YIELD: ABOUT 2 QUARTS (1.9 L)

Chicken stock, also called bone broth, is richer in flavor than broth, and I like it the best, but most of my recipes can be made with either broth or stock. I've read that adding a little acid to your chicken stock helps to draw out the nutrients—like collagen, gelatin, and minerals—from the bones, making it even more nutritious. So I always include a tablespoon (15 ml) of lemon juice or vinegar in mine. Not that doing this increases the fat content: There's so little fat in this stock that I rarely need to strain any of it off.

BONES OF 1 (2½- TO 4-POUND, OR 1.1 TO 1.8 KG) CHICKEN

10 CUPS (2.4 L) WATER

2 LARGE CARROTS, CUT INTO 1-INCH (2.5 CM) PIECES

1 STALK OF CELERY, CUT INTO 1-INCH (2.5 CM) PIECES (OR JUST USE THE LEAVES AND NOT THE STALKS IF YOU ARE SENSITIVE TO CELERY)

1 BUNCH OF SCALLIONS (GREEN PARTS ONLY), CUT INTO 1-INCH (2.5 CM) PIECES

6 SPRIGS OF FRESH ITALIAN PARSLEY

3 BAY LEAVES

¼ TEASPOON WHOLE BLACK PEPPERCORNS

1 TABLESPOON (15 ML) WHITE VINEGAR OR FRESH LEMON JUICE

Combine all of the ingredients in a large pot or Dutch oven. Bring to a boil over high heat. Reduce the heat to low, cover, and cook just under a simmer for at least 4 hours and up to 24 hours. (The longer it simmers, the better it is.) You can also do this in a slow cooker set to low heat.

Strain the stock through a fine-mesh sieve and discard the solids. Either use the stock right away, store in the fridge for a couple of days, or freeze in portions of different sizes so it's ready to be used in your favorite recipes.

CHICKEN BROTH

YIELD: ABOUT 4 QUARTS (3.8 L)

All soups and stews require some type of broth or stock as a base. But what's the difference? Well, according to Alton Brown, one of my food heroes, broths are liquids in which meat has been cooked, while stock is the liquid in which bones have been simmered. Homemade chicken broth is much better than the store-bought stuff, and it's worlds away from those grainy, processed cubes.

1 WHOLE CHICKEN (2½ TO 4 POUNDS, OR 1.1 TO 1.8 KG), GIBLETS AND NECK REMOVED

2 LARGE CARROTS, CUT INTO 1-INCH (2.5 CM) PIECES

1 STALK OF CELERY, CUT INTO 1-INCH (2.5 CM) PIECES (OR JUST USE THE LEAVES AND NOT THE STALKS IF YOU ARE SENSITIVE TO CELERY)

1 BUNCH OF SCALLIONS (GREEN PARTS ONLY), CUT INTO 1-INCH (2.5 CM) PIECES

6 SPRIGS OF FRESH ITALIAN PARSLEY

3 BAY LEAVES

¼ TEASPOON WHOLE BLACK PEPPERCORNS

Combine all of the ingredients in a large pot or Dutch oven. Add enough water to cover the chicken by a few inches (7.5 to 10 cm). Cover and bring to a boil over high heat. Reduce the heat to low, cover, and simmer for 1½ to 2 hours until the meat starts to fall off the bones.

Remove the chicken from the pot and when cool enough to handle, remove the chicken meat from the bones and set aside to use for soups or casseroles. Reserve the bones to make stock (page 109).

Strain the broth through a fine-mesh sieve and discard the solids. Let cool completely and then refrigerate until the fat solidifies on top. Skim the fat off the top and discard. Either use the broth right away, store in the fridge for a couple of days, or freeze in portions of different sizes so it's ready to be used in your favorite recipes.

Hold the salt. Notice that neither this Chicken Broth recipe nor the Chicken Stock recipe on page 109 call for salt? There's a reason: It means that I can add salt to taste when I'm using it in individual recipes.

BEEF STOCK

YIELD: ABOUT 2 QUARTS (1.9 L)

When it comes to beef stock, there's a simple trick that will ensure a rich, flavorful result: Roast the bones first. Roasting may require a little extra time, but the process is so simple, and it's worth it since the browned bits add such color and depth to the broth. Prepackaged soup bones can sometimes be found in the meat department of the grocery store. If you don't see them there, inquire at the meat counter.

3 TO 4 POUNDS (1.4 TO 1.8 KG) BEEF MARROW SOUP BONES

2 CARROTS, CUT INTO 1-INCH (2.5 CM) PIECES

½ CUP (120 ML) WATER

1 STALK OF CELERY, CUT INTO 1-INCH (2.5 CM) PIECES (OR JUST USE THE LEAVES AND NOT THE STALKS IF YOU ARE SENSITIVE TO CELERY)

1 BUNCH OF SCALLIONS (GREEN PARTS ONLY), CUT INTO 1-INCH (2.5 CM) PIECES

6 SPRIGS OF FRESH ITALIAN PARSLEY

3 BAY LEAVES

1 TABLESPOON (15 ML) VINEGAR

1 TEASPOON DRIED THYME OR 1 SPRIG FRESH

¼ TEASPOON WHOLE BLACK PEPPERCORNS

Preheat the oven to 450°F (230°C, or gas mark 8). Combine the bones and carrots in a large roasting pan. Bake, uncovered, for 30 minutes, turning the bones and carrots occasionally.

Using tongs, transfer the bones and carrots to a large stockpot. Drain the fat from the roasting pan and discard. Pour the ½ cup (120 ml) water into the roasting pan and scrape up the browned bits using a wooden spoon. Pour this into the stockpot as well.

Add all of the remaining ingredients to the stockpot and then add enough water to completely cover the bones. Bring to a boil over high heat and then reduce the heat to low. Cover and cook just below a simmer for 4 to 5 hours, or even longer if desired, adding more water if needed to keep the bones covered.

Strain the stock through a fine-mesh sieve or a colander lined with cheesecloth. Cool the stock and transfer it to the refrigerator. Let it chill overnight. Skim the solid fat off the top. Either use the stock right away, store in the fridge for a couple of days, or freeze in portions of different sizes so it's ready to be used in your favorite recipes.

VEGETABLE BROTH

YIELD: ABOUT 6 CUPS (1.4 L)

If you're vegetarian or vegan—or if you just don't have the time or resources to make bone broth—you can use this vegetable broth as a speedy stand-in. It takes just half an hour to make, and it's a vital ingredient in some of the recipes in this book, like the Salmon Chowder on page 118 and the Vegan Lentil Minestrone on page 120. Freeze leftover vegetable scraps for this: Things like carrot peels and celery leaves are perfect for making broths.

1 TABLESPOON (15 ML) OLIVE OIL

1 CLOVE OF GARLIC, PEELED AND SMASHED, BUT KEPT WHOLE

2 LARGE CARROTS, CUT INTO 1-INCH (2.5 CM) PIECES

1 STALK OF CELERY, CUT INTO 1-INCH (2.5 CM) PIECES (OR JUST USE THE LEAVES AND NOT THE STALKS IF YOU ARE SENSITIVE TO CELERY)

2 CUPS (178 G) COARSELY CHOPPED LEEKS (GREEN PARTS ONLY)

8 CUPS (1.9 L) WATER

½ OF A BUNCH OF SCALLIONS (GREEN PARTS ONLY), SLICED INTO 1-INCH (2.5 CM) PIECES

6 SPRIGS OF FRESH ITALIAN PARSLEY

6 SPRIGS OF FRESH THYME

3 BAY LEAVES

¼ TEASPOON WHOLE PEPPERCORNS

Heat the oil in a large stockpot over medium-high heat. Sauté the garlic until browned. Remove and discard. Add the carrots, celery, and leeks. Cook, stirring occasionally, until lightly browned, about 6 to 8 minutes.

Add the water, scallions, fresh parsley, fresh thyme, bay leaves, and peppercorns. Bring to a boil and then reduce the heat and simmer, uncovered, for about 30 minutes.

Pour the broth through a fine-mesh sieve and discard the solids. Either use the broth right away, store in the fridge for a couple of days, or freeze in portions of different sizes so it's ready to be used in your favorite recipes.

CHICKEN SOUP, THREE WAYS

YIELD: 6 TO 8 SERVINGS EACH

Nothing beats a bowl of classic chicken soup—like this low-FODMAP version—especially if you're a bit under the weather. But chicken soup is so versatile that I couldn't resist coming up with a couple of variations on the theme! My Herbed Basmati Rice Chicken Soup is fragrant with thyme, basil, chives, and rosemary, while the Lemon Chicken Quinoa Soup sports the bright flavors of cumin and fresh lemon. All of these soups make great light lunches or dinners: Serve them with Mom's Best Biscuits (page 76) or Maple Cinnamon Corn Bread (page 77).

CLASSIC CHICKEN NOODLE SOUP

8 CUPS (1.9 L) CHICKEN STOCK OR CHICKEN BROTH (PAGE 109 OR 110)

2 CUPS (280 G) SHREDDED COOKED CHICKEN

1 CUP (130 G) SLICED CARROTS (ABOUT 3 LARGE)

1 STALK OF CELERY, SLICED

1 CUP (112 G) GLUTEN-FREE FUSILLI PASTA

½ TEASPOON DRIED OREGANO

½ TEASPOON DRIED BASIL

1½ TEASPOONS KOSHER SALT (OR TO TASTE)

½ TEASPOON FRESHLY GROUND BLACK PEPPER

Bring the chicken stock or broth to a boil in a large stockpot or Dutch oven. Add the shredded chicken, carrots, celery, pasta, oregano, basil, kosher salt, and black pepper. Reduce the heat and simmer for 15 minutes or until the vegetables and pasta are tender. Serve hot.

HERBED BASMATI RICE CHICKEN SOUP

Follow the directions for Classic Chicken Noodle Soup, but make the following changes:

REPLACE THE PASTA WITH ½ CUP (96 G) LONG-GRAIN BASMATI RICE.

REPLACE THE OREGANO WITH DRIED THYME.

INCREASE THE BASIL TO 1 TEASPOON.

ADD 1 TEASPOON DRIED CHIVES.

ADD ¼ TEASPOON CRUSHED DRIED ROSEMARY.

LEMON CHICKEN QUINOA SOUP

Follow the directions for Classic Chicken Noodle Soup, but make the following changes:

REPLACE THE PASTA WITH ½ CUP (87 G) RINSED QUINOA.

OMIT THE CELERY, BASIL, AND OREGANO.

ADD 2 TEASPOONS GROUND CUMIN AND ¼ CUP (60 ML) FRESH LEMON JUICE.

JUST BEFORE SERVING, ADD 2 CUPS (60 G) FRESH BABY SPINACH AND STIR UNTIL WILTED.

CREAMY HAM AND POTATO SOUP

YIELD: 4 TO 6 SERVINGS

For wintertime comfort food, you can't do better than this hearty soup, especially if you're saddled with leftovers (after the holidays, perhaps?) and have lots of extra ham on hand. Use tender-skinned red potatoes and leave them unpeeled: Peeling them strips them of some of their fiber and nutrients. This recipe was inspired by a similar one on allrecipes.com.

1½ POUNDS (680 G) RED POTATOES, DICED INTO ¾-INCH (2 CM) CUBES (ABOUT 4½ CUPS)

1 STALK OF CELERY, SLICED

2 CUPS (300 G) DICED COOKED HAM

4 CUPS (946 ML) CHICKEN BROTH OR CHICKEN STOCK (PAGE 110 OR 109)

4 TABLESPOONS (55 G) UNSALTED BUTTER OR MARGARINE

3 TABLESPOONS (30 G) BASIC FLOUR BLEND (PAGE 38)

1½ CUPS (355 ML) LACTOSE-FREE OR NONDAIRY MILK

1 TEASPOON KOSHER SALT (OR TO TASTE)

½ TEASPOON FRESHLY GROUND BLACK PEPPER

4 SCALLIONS (GREEN PARTS ONLY), SLICED

Place the potatoes, celery, diced ham, and chicken broth or stock in a large stockpot or Dutch oven and bring to a boil. Reduce the heat to medium or medium-low and simmer for about 15 minutes or until the potatoes and celery are tender. (You'll need a good simmer to cook the potatoes and celery, but try not to simmer so vigorously that all the liquid gets cooked off.)

Meanwhile, melt the butter in a medium saucepan over medium heat. Stir in the Basic Flour Blend. Slowly add the milk while constantly stirring. Continue cooking and stirring over medium heat for a few minutes or until the mixture has thickened.

Once the potatoes and celery are tender, slowly add the butter mixture, while stirring. Season the soup with the kosher salt and black pepper and serve hot, topped with the sliced scallions.

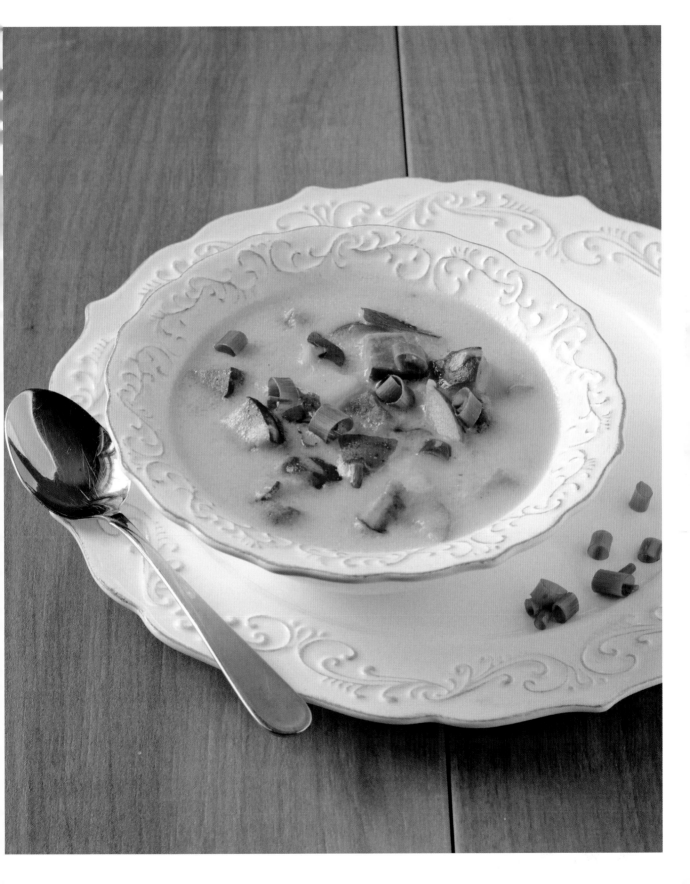

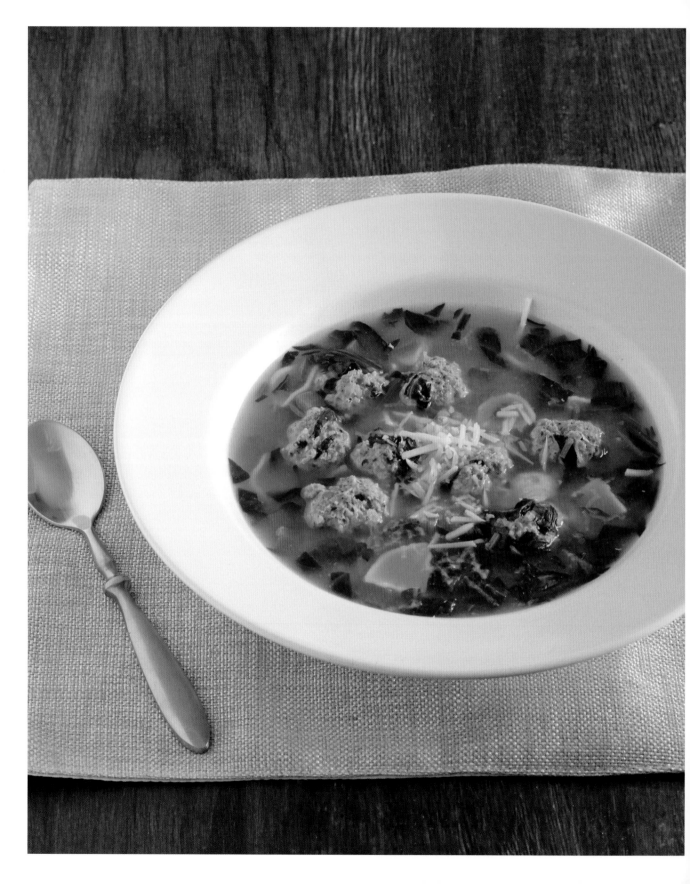

ITALIAN WEDDING SOUP

YIELD: 4 TO 6 SERVINGS

Italian wedding soup is traditionally made with orzo pasta, but since I have yet to find a gluten-free orzo pasta, I like to use gluten-free pasta shells instead. (Rice is a great alternative, too.) This low-FODMAP take on the original calls for ground turkey, but really, any kind of ground meat would be lovely here. And if you're sensitive to eggs, use a Chia Egg Replacer (page 39) instead of a regular one; it will bind the miniature meatballs just as well.

1 POUND (455 G) GROUND BEEF, CHICKEN, OR TURKEY

½ CUP (51 G) QUINOA FLAKES, QUICK-COOKING OATS (40 G), OR BREAD CRUMBS (60 G) (PAGE 73)

½ OF A BUNCH OF SCALLIONS (GREEN PARTS ONLY), SLICED

1 LARGE EGG OR 1 CHIA EGG REPLACER (PAGE 39)

1 TEASPOON DRIED BASIL

1½ TEASPOONS KOSHER SALT (OR TO TASTE), DIVIDED

¼ TEASPOON FRESHLY GROUND BLACK PEPPER

8 CUPS (946 ML) CHICKEN BROTH OR CHICKEN STOCK (PAGE 110 OR 109)

1 CUP (112 G) SMALL GLUTEN-FREE PASTA (SUCH AS SHELLS), OR ⅓ CUP (64 G) RICE

1 CUP (130 G) FINELY CHOPPED CARROTS

3 CUPS (90 G) CHOPPED FRESH BABY SPINACH

GRATED PARMESAN CHEESE, FOR SERVING

In the bowl of a stand mixer, blend together the ground meat, quinoa flakes, scallions, egg, basil, ½ teaspoon of the kosher salt, and black pepper. Shape into ¾-inch (2 cm) balls (about ½ tablespoonful of the mixture for each meatball).

In a large stockpot or Dutch oven, bring the chicken broth or stock to a boil. Stir in the meatballs, pasta, and carrots. Reduce the heat and simmer, stirring frequently, until the pasta and carrots are tender and the meatballs are cooked through, about 15 minutes.

Stir in the remaining 1½ teaspoons kosher salt, or to taste, and the spinach. Simmer just until the spinach is wilted. Serve sprinkled with Parmesan cheese.

SALMON CHOWDER

YIELD: 4 SERVINGS

With its abundance of protein, omega-3s, and essential vitamins, salmon is truly a superfood, and this chowder is such an easy, inexpensive way to fit it into your diet. Plus, it's uncomplicated enough to make on a weeknight—and that's a huge bonus, if you ask me! Serve it with a hunk of Maple Cinnamon Cornbread (page 77).

1 TABLESPOON (15 ML) OLIVE OIL

1 CLOVE OF GARLIC, PEELED AND SMASHED, BUT KEPT WHOLE

1 STALK OF CELERY, CHOPPED

2 CUPS (475 ML) CHICKEN STOCK, VEGETABLE BROTH, OR CHICKEN BROTH (PAGE 109, 112, OR 110)

2 CUPS (475 ML) LACTOSE-FREE OR NONDAIRY MILK

¾ POUND (340 G) RED POTATOES, DICED (ABOUT 2 CUPS)

2 CARROTS, CHOPPED (ABOUT ¾ CUP, OR 98 G)

1 TEASPOON KOSHER SALT

¼ TEASPOON FRESHLY GROUND BLACK PEPPER

¼ CUP (60 ML) WATER

2 TABLESPOONS (20 G) BASIC FLOUR BLEND (PAGE 38)

2 POUCHES (5 OUNCES EACH, OR 140 G) BONELESS, SKINLESS PINK SALMON, FLAKED

2 TEASPOONS CHOPPED FRESH DILL

Heat the olive oil in a large stockpot or Dutch oven over medium heat. Add the garlic and sauté for 1½ to 2 minutes, removing and discarding the garlic before it becomes too brown. Add the celery and sauté until slightly softened, about 3 minutes. Add the stock or broth, milk, potatoes, carrots, kosher salt, and black pepper. Raise the heat to high and bring to a boil. Reduce the heat and simmer, uncovered, for about 20 minutes or until the potatoes and carrots are tender.

Measure the water using a small glass measuring cup. Stir in the Basic Flour Blend and stir until smooth. Slowly pour the flour mixture into the chowder, while constantly stirring. Continue cooking for about 5 minutes or until thickened.

Stir in the flaked salmon and chopped fresh dill and cook until just heated through. Serve hot.

SLOW COOKER BEEF STEW

YIELD: 8 SERVINGS

As a Midwesterner, I've learned to embrace the slow cooker. And this is probably my favorite slow cooker recipe of all time: I make it at least monthly once the weather turns cold. Since it makes enough to serve eight people, you're sure to have plenty of leftovers to help stock up your freezer (unless you have dinner guests or a big family). Either way, be sure to serve it with the Mom's Best Biscuits on page 76. It's pure comfort food, through and through.

1½ POUNDS (680 G) RED POTATOES, CUBED

4 MEDIUM CARROTS, PEELED AND COARSELY CHOPPED

2 STALKS OF CELERY, COARSELY CHOPPED

1 BUNCH OF SCALLIONS (GREEN PARTS ONLY), CUT INTO 1-INCH (2.5 CM) PIECES

1 TEASPOON DRIED PARSLEY

1 TEASPOON CRUSHED DRIED ROSEMARY

½ TEASPOON DRIED THYME

4 CUPS (946 ML) BEEF STOCK (PAGE 111)

2 POUNDS (910 G) BEEF STEW MEAT, CUT INTO 1-INCH (2.5 CM) CUBES

4 TABLESPOONS (41 G) BASIC FLOUR BLEND (PAGE 38), DIVIDED

1 TEASPOON KOSHER SALT

½ TEASPOON FRESHLY GROUND BLACK PEPPER

2 TABLESPOONS (28 ML) OLIVE OIL

½ CUP (120 ML) DRY RED WINE OR BEEF STOCK (PAGE 111)

¼ CUP (60 ML) WATER

Place the potatoes, carrots, celery, scallions, parsley, rosemary, thyme, and beef stock in a large slow cooker.

Place the beef cubes, 2 tablespoons (20 g) of the Basic Flour Blend, kosher salt, and black pepper in a large resealable plastic bag. Shake to coat the beef. Heat the olive oil in a large skillet over medium-high heat. Add the beef and brown on all sides, working in batches so as to not crowd the skillet. Transfer the beef to the slow cooker. Deglaze the skillet by adding the red wine or additional beef stock and scraping up the browned bits. Pour this into the slow cooker as well.

Stir well to combine all the ingredients in the slow cooker. Cook on the high setting for 4 to 6 hours or on the low setting for 10 to 12 hours.

About 30 minutes before serving, combine the ¼ cup water (60 ml) and remaining 2 tablespoons (20 g) Basic Flour Blend in a small bowl and then gradually add to the stew, while stirring. Cook for 30 minutes on high or until thickened. Serve hot.

VEGAN LENTIL MINESTRONE

YIELD: 6 SERVINGS

Through my research on diet and nutrition, I've really come to appreciate the wisdom of eating less animal protein. Not only is it better for your health, but it's also better for the environment. Enter this flavorful vegan version! It's one of my lunchtime staples, and it's got a healthy balance of protein, fiber, and vegetables. And, of course, it's low-FODMAP, too. It's an all-round winner.

1 TABLESPOON (15 ML) OLIVE OIL

½ CUP (60 G) CHOPPED ZUCCHINI

1 STALK OF CELERY, MINCED

4 SCALLIONS (GREEN PARTS ONLY), THINLY SLICED

6 CUPS (1.4 L) VEGETABLE BROTH (PAGE 112)

1 CAN (14 OUNCES, OR 390 G) NO-SALT-ADDED DICED TOMATOES

½ CUP (65 G) CHOPPED CARROT

1 TEASPOON DRIED BASIL

1 TEASPOON DRIED OREGANO

1½ TEASPOONS KOSHER SALT (OR TO TASTE)

½ TEASPOON FRESHLY GROUND BLACK PEPPER

1 CAN (14 OUNCES, OR 390 G) LENTILS, RINSED AND DRAINED

1 CUP (112 G) BROWN RICE PASTA SHELLS

Heat the olive oil in a large stockpot or Dutch oven over medium heat. Add the zucchini, celery, and scallions and sauté until the vegetables are tender, about 5 minutes.

Stir in the vegetable broth, diced tomatoes, carrots, basil, oregano, kosher salt, and black pepper. Raise the heat to high and bring to a boil. Reduce the heat to medium and simmer for 10 minutes.

Add the lentils and pasta. Raise the heat to medium-high and continue simmering until the pasta is tender, about 15 to 20 minutes.

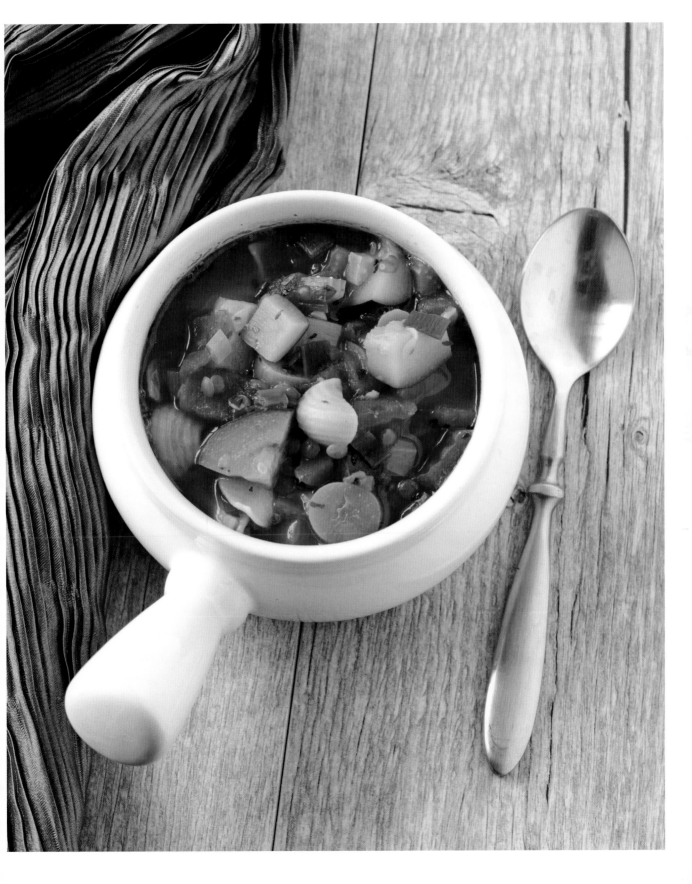

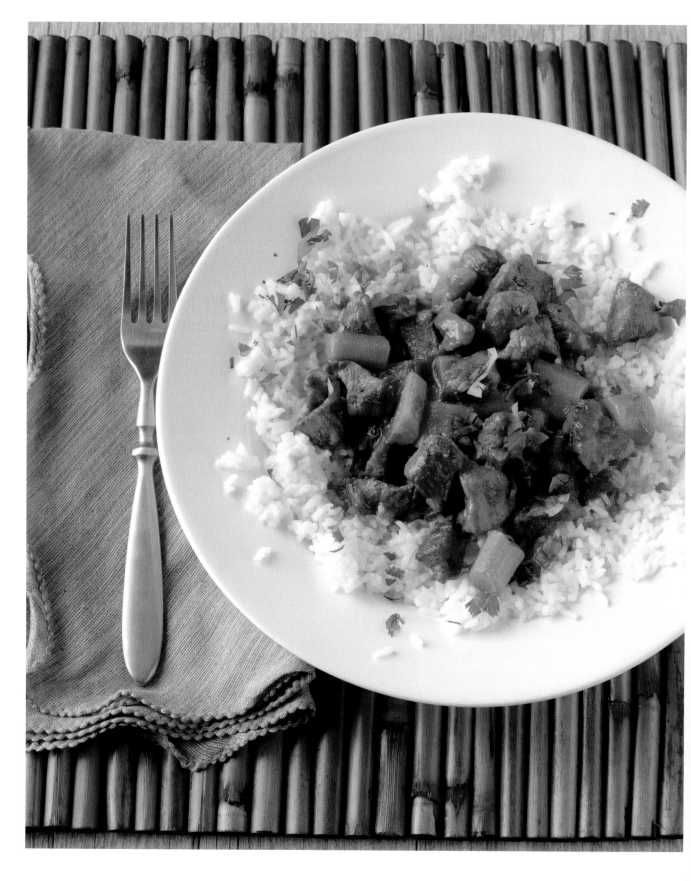

CURRIED LAMB STEW

YIELD: 4 SERVINGS

My husband and I first tried lamb stew just a couple of years ago, and now we love it. Lamb works perfectly with the Indian-inspired spices featured in this recipe (but if you're not a fan of lamb, beef works just as well). Coriander adds a wonderful earthiness to the dish. Spoon this stew over basmati rice.

1 POUND (455 G) LAMB (OR BEEF) STEW MEAT, CUT INTO 1-INCH (2.5 CM) CUBES

1 TEASPOON KOSHER SALT

½ TEASPOON FRESHLY GROUND BLACK PEPPER

2 TABLESPOONS (20 G) BASIC FLOUR BLEND (PAGE 38), DIVIDED

2 TABLESPOONS (28 ML) OLIVE OIL

1 CLOVE OF GARLIC

1½ CUPS (355 ML) BEEF STOCK (PAGE 111)

1 TEASPOON GROUND CORIANDER

½ TEASPOON GROUND CUMIN

¼ TEASPOON GROUND GINGER

¼ TEASPOON GROUND TURMERIC

⅛ TEASPOON GROUND CINNAMON

PINCH OF GROUND RED CHILE PEPPER (OPTIONAL)

2 CARROTS, PEELED AND CHOPPED INTO 1-INCH (2.5 CM) PIECES

1 BUNCH OF SCALLIONS (GREEN PARTS ONLY), SLICED

1 TABLESPOON (15 ML) WATER

STEAMED BASMATI RICE, FOR SERVING

½ CUP (8 G) CHOPPED FRESH CILANTRO OR ITALIAN PARSLEY

Toss the lamb with the kosher salt, black pepper, and 1 tablespoon (10 g) of the Basic Flour Blend in a large resealable plastic bag.

Heat the olive oil in a large stockpot or Dutch oven over medium-high heat. Add the garlic and sauté until it starts to brown. Remove the garlic from the skillet and discard. Add the stew meat to the pot and brown on all sides. Remove the meat from the pot and drain any excess fat. Wipe the pot clean with a paper towel. Return the meat to the pot and stir in the beef stock, coriander (if using), cumin, ginger, turmeric, cinnamon, and red pepper (if using). Bring to a boil, reduce the heat to low, and simmer covered for 30 minutes.

Add the carrots and scallions and simmer covered for 30 minutes more or until the meat and carrots are tender.

In a small bowl, combine the remaining 1 tablespoon (10 g) Basic Flour Blend with the 1 tablespoon (15 ml) water. Pour this flour mixture into the stew, while constantly stirring. Cook for a few minutes until thickened and bubbly. Season with more kosher salt and black pepper, if desired.

Serve hot over basmati rice and garnish with chopped fresh cilantro or parsley.

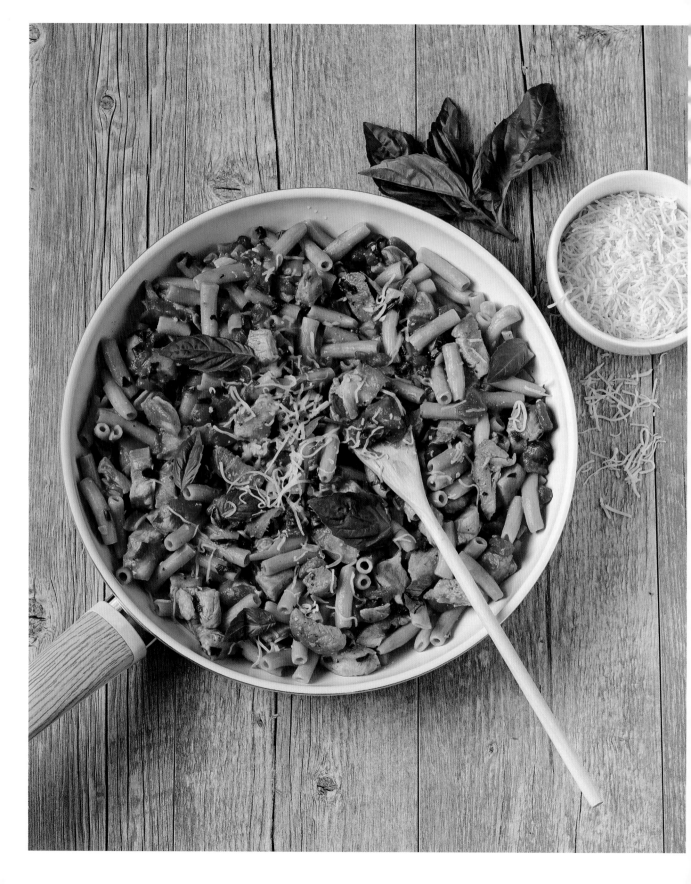

MAIN DISHES

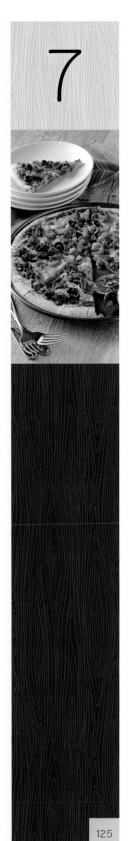

7

"What's for dinner?" It's a question we all have to grapple with every single day, whether we're cooking for one, two, or a crowd. And it's not always easy to find the answer, especially if you're on a low-FODMAP diet. Thankfully, this chapter is here to help. It's packed with stick-to-your-ribs Midwestern classics, like casseroles, roasts, and grilled meats, which are great when the weather turns sharp and chilly. (I'm an Iowa gal at heart, that's for sure!) But I also love healthy, lower-fat meals inspired by Italian, Asian, and Indian cuisine that feature lots of fresh vegetables, and you'll find those dishes here, too. Some of them are vegetarian or vegan and feature tempeh and tofu, which are both excellent meat-free, low-FODMAP protein choices. And you can rest assured that none of these dishes skimp on flavor. Once they're on the table, you'll forget that they're low-FODMAP and focus on how fabulous they taste.

All of these recipes are pretty quick and easy to make, but a little advance preparation can make things even simpler. If you've got frozen portions of chicken broth, vegetable broth, and pesto on hand (you can find the recipes for them in Chapters 3 and 6), you'll be a step ahead of the game when it comes to the daily dinner rush!

LEMON AND THYME ROAST CHICKEN

YIELD: 6 SERVINGS

It looks so impressive when it's done (and it fills the kitchen with such amazing aromas while it's in the oven!), but roast chicken is ridiculously easy to make. My version is loaded with lemon and fresh thyme, which bring out the crispiness of the skin and enhance the juicy flavor of the meat. Serve it with mashed potatoes and a salad and then take advantage of the leftovers: Make the Chicken Salad with Pecans and Grapes on page 86 and use the bones to make the Chicken Stock on page 109.

1 WHOLE CHICKEN (3½ TO 4 POUNDS, OR 1.6 TO 1.8 KG)

1 LEMON, QUARTERED LENGTHWISE

HANDFUL OF FRESH THYME SPRIGS (ABOUT 12 SPRIGS)

2 TEASPOONS KOSHER SALT

1 TEASPOON FRESHLY GROUND BLACK PEPPER

CHOPPED FRESH THYME LEAVES, FOR SERVING (OPTIONAL)

Preheat the oven to 375°F (190°C, or gas mark 5). Remove any giblets from the cavity of the chicken and discard them (or use them however you wish). Thoroughly dry the chicken with paper towels. Place the chicken breast side up in a large roasting pan.

Place 3 of the lemon quarters and the thyme sprigs in the cavity of the chicken. Tie the legs together with kitchen twine. Rub the kosher salt and black pepper all over the outside of the chicken. Tuck the wing tips up and under the neck.

Roast for about 1 hour 30 minutes or until the chicken reaches an internal temperature of 165°F (74°C); you can determine the temperature by inserting a kitchen thermometer into the thickest part of the thigh, being sure not to hit any bone. Remove the chicken from the oven and let it rest for about 15 minutes.

Squeeze the remaining lemon wedge over the cooked chicken before carving and sprinkle with chopped fresh thyme, if you like.

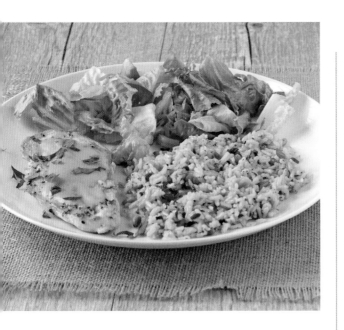

SAUTÉED CHICKEN WITH DIJON SAUCE

YIELD: 4 SERVINGS

Do you need a low-FODMAP weeknight meal that won't take forever to make? Whip up this Sautéed Chicken with Dijon Sauce: While you're at it, roast some potatoes in the oven, toss a salad, and dinner is served! There is one caveat, though: Be sure to check the label on your jar of Dijon mustard for FODMAP ingredients, like onion powder.

2 BONELESS, SKINLESS CHICKEN BREASTS (1 POUND, OR 455 G)

½ TEASPOON KOSHER SALT

½ TEASPOON FRESHLY GROUND BLACK PEPPER

1 TABLESPOON (15 ML) OLIVE OIL

¼ CUP (60 ML) DRY WHITE WINE

1 TABLESPOON (14 G) UNSALTED BUTTER

2 TEASPOONS BASIC FLOUR BLEND (PAGE 38)

¾ CUP (175 ML) CHICKEN BROTH OR CHICKEN STOCK (PAGE 110 OR 109)

1 TABLESPOON (15 G) DIJON MUSTARD

2 TABLESPOONS (8 G) CHOPPED FRESH ITALIAN PARSLEY

Fillet the chicken breasts by slicing them in half, holding the knife parallel to the counter. Season them with the kosher salt and black pepper. Heat the olive oil in a large skillet over medium-high heat. Add the chicken breasts to the skillet and cook until golden brown on the bottom, about 3 minutes, and then flip and reduce the heat to medium-low. Continue cooking until the chicken has reached an internal temperature of 165°F (74°C), about 3 to 4 minutes. Transfer to a plate and cover with aluminum foil to keep warm.

Remove the skillet from the heat and carefully deglaze it with the white wine, scraping up the brown bits on the bottom. Return the skillet to the heat, add the butter, and let it melt. Stir in the Basic Flour Blend to form a roux. Slowly whisk in the chicken broth or stock, stirring out any lumps. Simmer for about 5 minutes or until the liquid is reduced by half. Stir in the Dijon mustard. Season with kosher salt and black pepper to taste, if desired.

Spoon the Dijon sauce over the chicken, sprinkle with the chopped fresh parsley, and serve.

OVEN-FRIED CHICKEN FINGERS WITH MAPLE MUSTARD DIPPING SAUCE

YIELD: 4 SERVINGS

Kids and grown-ups alike will love these homemade chicken fingers served with a sweet-and-savory dipping sauce that takes about two seconds to stir together. Soaking the chicken in a "buttermilk" bath of lactose-free milk and lemon juice keeps them moist and tender on the inside, while low-FODMAP gluten-free cornflakes add a satisfying crunch. (If cornflakes aren't your thing, though, you can use crushed crispy rice cereal or gluten-free cracker crumbs—or a combination of any of these items—instead.) All you need on the side here is a fresh green salad. This recipe was inspired by *Cooking Light* magazine.

1 POUND (455 G) BONELESS, SKINLESS CHICKEN TENDERS

½ CUP (120 ML) LACTOSE-FREE OR NONDAIRY MILK

2 TEASPOONS FRESH LEMON JUICE

1 CUP (34 G) CRUSHED GLUTEN-FREE CORNFLAKES, GLUTEN-FREE CRUSHED CRISPY RICE CEREAL (34 G), OR CRUSHED GLUTEN-FREE CRACKERS (25 G)

1 TEASPOON DRIED OREGANO

½ TEASPOON KOSHER SALT

¼ TEASPOON FRESHLY GROUND BLACK PEPPER

¼ CUP (60 G) MAYONNAISE

2 TABLESPOONS (30 G) DIJON MUSTARD

1 TO 2 TABLESPOONS (15 TO 28 ML) PURE MAPLE SYRUP

Preheat the oven to 400°F (200°C, or gas mark 6). Spray a large baking sheet with olive oil cooking spray. (For easy cleanup, line the sheet with aluminum foil first.)

Place the chicken tenders in a shallow glass baking dish. Combine the milk and lemon juice and pour over the chicken. Cover and refrigerate for 10 to 15 minutes, flipping the chicken tenders over halfway through.

On a shallow plate, combine the cornflake crumbs, oregano, kosher salt, and black pepper. Remove the chicken tenders from the milk mixture, draining off any excess liquid. Roll each chicken tender in the cornflake mixture to coat evenly. Place the chicken tenders on the prepared baking sheet. Bake for 8 minutes. Turn the chicken tenders over and bake for another 7 to 9 minutes until they're no longer pink inside and the juices run clear.

While the chicken is baking, prepare the dipping sauce by stirring the mayonnaise and Dijon mustard together in a small bowl until smooth. Whisk in the maple syrup to taste. Serve the chicken fingers with the dipping sauce.

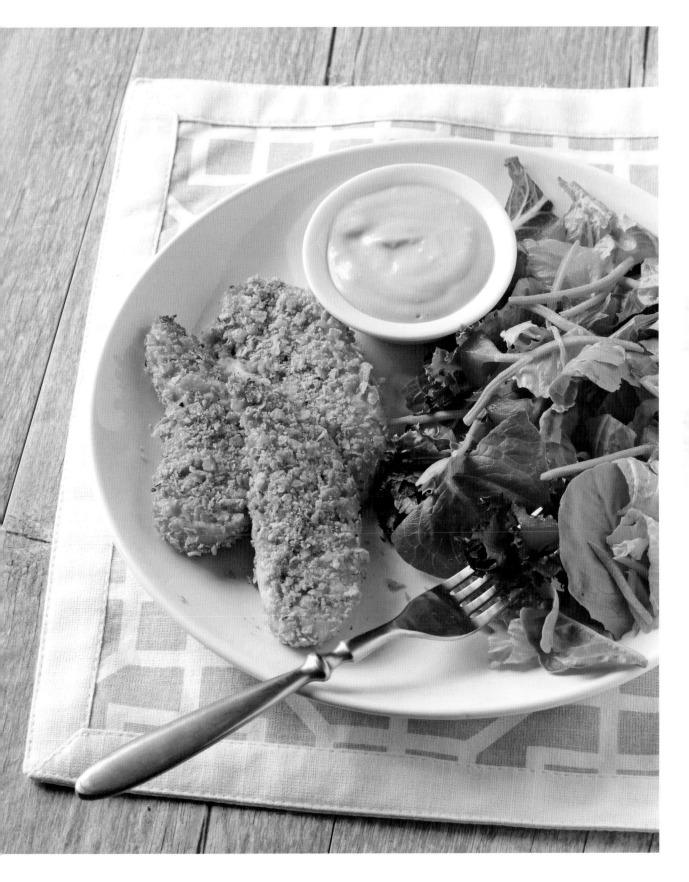

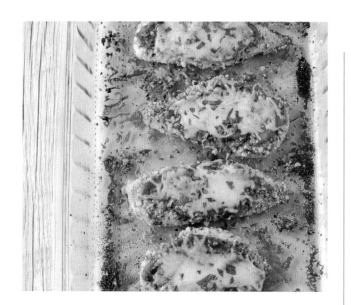

WALNUT-CRUSTED CHICKEN PARMESAN

YIELD: 4 SERVINGS

This classic recipe gets a wheat-free makeover when you use finely chopped walnuts to "bread" the chicken—and since the chicken is baked instead of fried, it's healthier and lower in fat than the traditional version. Serve it with the Caesar Salad on page 83.

¼ CUP (30 G) FINELY CHOPPED WALNUTS

¼ CUP (25 G) GRATED PARMESAN CHEESE

1 TEASPOON ITALIAN HERB SEASONING (PAGE 40)

¼ TEASPOON KOSHER SALT

¼ TEASPOON FRESHLY GROUND BLACK PEPPER

4 THIN BONELESS, SKINLESS CHICKEN BREASTS (1 TO 1½ POUNDS, OR 455 TO 680 G)

1 TABLESPOON (14 G) UNSALTED BUTTER, MELTED

¼ CUP (60 ML) CLASSIC TOMATO PIZZA SAUCE (PAGE 164)

¼ CUP (30 G) SHREDDED MOZZARELLA CHEESE

Preheat the oven to 400°F (200°C, or gas mark 6). Spray a 9 x 13-inch (23 x 33 cm) baking pan with cooking spray.

Combine the chopped walnuts, Parmesan cheese, Italian herb seasoning, kosher salt, and black pepper in a small bowl. Spread the mixture out on a plate.

Lightly brush each chicken breast with the melted butter and then dip them into the chopped walnut mixture, lightly pressing down so that the walnut "crumbs" stick. Place the chicken in the baking pan. Sprinkle any remaining mixture over the top. Bake for 25 to 30 minutes until the chicken is cooked through and lightly browned. Remove from the oven, spread each breast with a tablespoon (15 ml) of the Classic Tomato Pizza Sauce, and sprinkle evenly with the shredded mozzarella cheese. Bake for 5 more minutes or until the cheese is melted. Serve hot.

SLOW COOKER LEMON OLIVE CHICKEN

YIELD: 4 SERVINGS

When it comes to meat-based mains, your slow cooker should be your best friend. It does all the hard work for you—and plus, slow-cooked meat is fall-off-the-bone tender. Use chicken thighs instead of breasts in this recipe since they stay so moist in the slow cooker. When dinner's ready, spoon the chicken with its lemon-and-olive-laden sauce over basmati rice and serve with a side salad.

1½ POUNDS (680 G) BONELESS, SKINLESS CHICKEN THIGHS

½ TEASPOON KOSHER SALT

½ TEASPOON FRESHLY GROUND BLACK PEPPER

1 TABLESPOON (15 ML) OLIVE OIL

1 CLOVE OF GARLIC, PEELED AND SMASHED, BUT KEPT WHOLE

¼ CUP (60 ML) DRY WHITE WINE OR CHICKEN BROTH

1½ CUPS (355 ML) CHICKEN STOCK OR CHICKEN BROTH (PAGE 109 OR 110)

½ TEASPOON GRATED LEMON ZEST

2 TABLESPOONS (28 ML) FRESH LEMON JUICE

2 TEASPOONS DRIED BASIL

1 TEASPOON DRIED OREGANO

½ CUP (85 G) KALAMATA OLIVES, PITTED, DRAINED, AND HALVED

2 TABLESPOONS (20 G) BASIC FLOUR BLEND (PAGE 38)

¼ CUP (60 ML) WATER

COOKED BASMATI RICE, FOR SERVING

¼ CUP (15 G) CHOPPED FRESH ITALIAN PARSLEY

Season the chicken thighs with the kosher salt and black pepper. Heat the olive oil in a large skillet over medium-high heat. Add the garlic and sauté until fragrant, about 1 minute. Remove the garlic from the skillet and discard. Add the chicken to the skillet and brown it, about 3 to 4 minutes per side. Transfer the chicken to the slow cooker. Deglaze the skillet by adding the white wine or chicken broth to the skillet and scraping up any brown bits on the bottom. Pour this mixture into the slow cooker, onto the chicken.

In a medium bowl, combine the chicken stock or broth, lemon zest, lemon juice, basil, and oregano and pour the mixture over the chicken. Sprinkle with the Kalamata olives. Cover and cook on the low setting for 7 to 8 hours or on the high setting for 3 to 4 hours.

When the chicken is done, make a slurry by stirring the Basic Flour Blend and water together in a small bowl. Slowly pour into the liquid in the slow cooker, while constantly stirring. Turn the slow cooker to high. Continue cooking for about 10 minutes or until the sauce is thickened. The chicken will be very tender, and you can break it apart into smaller pieces, if desired. Season to taste with kosher salt and black pepper. Serve over basmati rice and sprinkle with the chopped fresh parsley.

CHICKEN PENNE IN TOMATO AND BASIL CREAM SAUCE

YIELD: 4 SERVINGS

Quick and easy enough for a weeknight meal but elegant and delicious enough for company, this chicken and pasta dish is sure to become one of your favorites. Since cream contains lactose, I've replaced it with a mixture of lactose-free milk and my Basic Flour Blend, which thickens it up nicely.

2 CUPS (224 G) GLUTEN-FREE BROWN RICE PENNE PASTA

1 TABLESPOON (15 ML) OLIVE OIL

1 CLOVE OF GARLIC, PEELED AND SMASHED, BUT KEPT WHOLE

1 POUND (455 G) BONELESS, SKINLESS CHICKEN BREASTS, CUT INTO 1-INCH (2.5 CM) CUBES

1 TEASPOON KOSHER SALT, DIVIDED

1 TEASPOON FRESHLY GROUND BLACK PEPPER, DIVIDED

1 TABLESPOON (14 G) UNSALTED BUTTER

½ OF A BUNCH OF SCALLIONS (GREEN PARTS ONLY), SLICED

1 CAN (14½ OUNCES, OR 410 G) UNSALTED DICED TOMATOES, UNDRAINED

½ CUP (20 G) CHOPPED FRESH BASIL, OR 1 TABLESPOON (2 G) DRIED

½ CUP (120 ML) LACTOSE-FREE MILK

2 TEASPOONS BASIC FLOUR BLEND (PAGE 38)

¼ CUP (25 G) GRATED PARMESAN CHEESE

Cook the pasta according to the package directions. Drain into a colander and rinse with cold water. Drain again.

While the pasta is cooking, heat the olive oil in a large skillet over medium-high heat. Add the garlic and cook until it starts to sizzle. Continue to cook for 1½ to 2 minutes more or just until the garlic starts to brown. Remove the garlic and discard.

Season the chicken with ½ teaspoon each of the kosher salt and black pepper. Add the chicken to the hot skillet and sauté over medium-high heat until browned and cooked through, about 6 to 8 minutes. Transfer the chicken to a plate and set aside.

Reduce the heat to medium and melt the butter. Add the scallions and cook until tender, about 1 minute. Add the tomatoes and basil and then increase the heat to medium-high. Simmer until the liquid is almost all absorbed, about 2 minutes.

In a small bowl, combine the milk and Basic Flour Blend, stirring until smooth. Slowly pour the milk mixture into the skillet, while stirring constantly. Continue to cook and stir until thickened. Stir in the cooked pasta and chicken and cook until heated through. Season with the remaining ½ teaspoon each kosher salt and black pepper. Serve sprinkled with the Parmesan cheese.

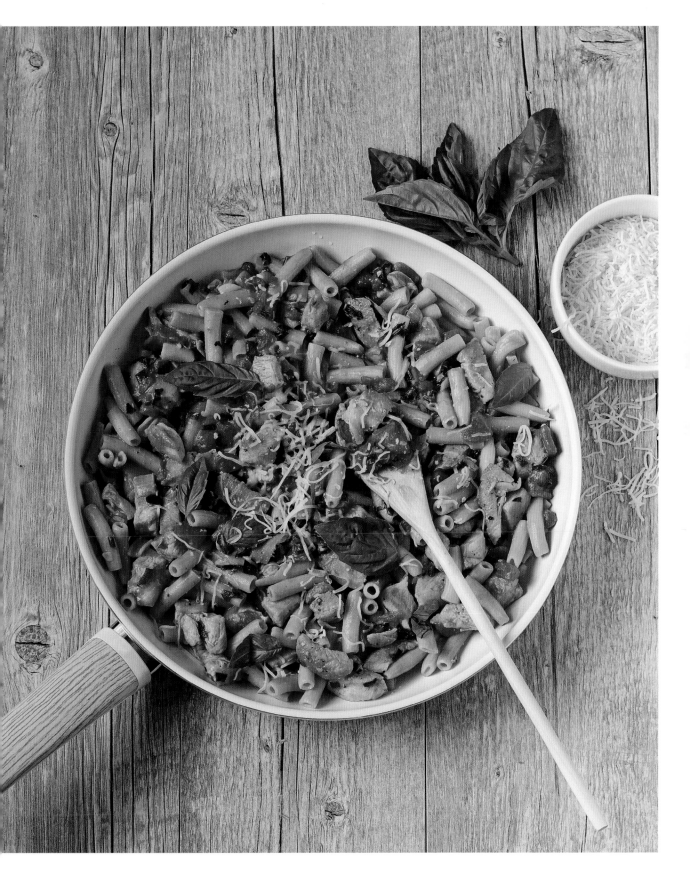

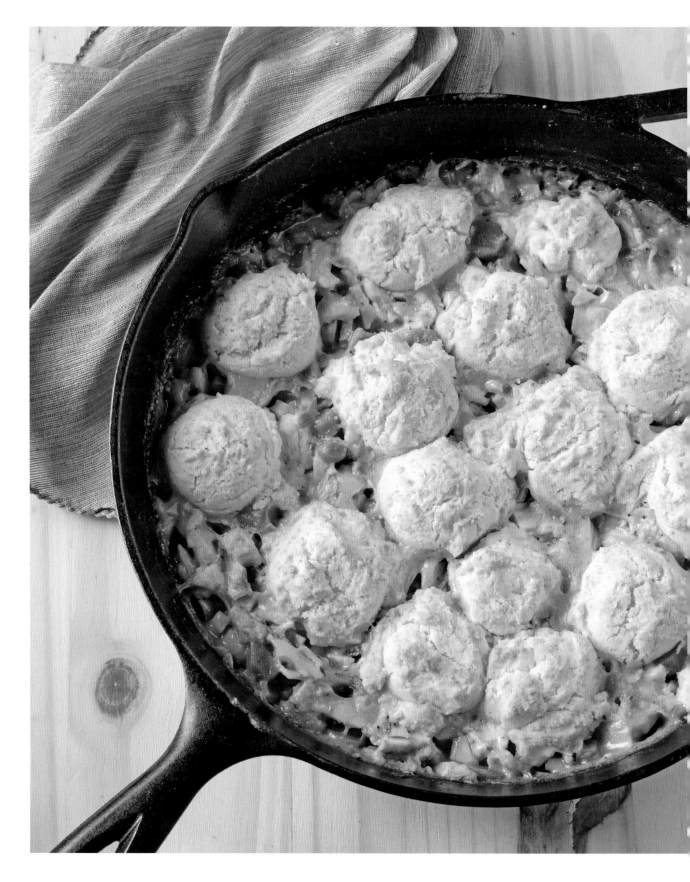

SKILLET CHICKEN POT PIE

YIELD: 4 SERVINGS

This low-FODMAP pot pie is the antidote to the cold-weather blues. It's hearty and substantial, but if you prefer something with less fat, you can serve the chicken filling over steamed rice or gluten-free pasta in place of the biscuit crust.

Biscuit Topping

1½ CUPS (243 G) BASIC FLOUR BLEND (PAGE 38)

2 TEASPOONS SUGAR

1 TEASPOON BAKING POWDER

½ TEASPOON KOSHER SALT

4 TABLESPOONS (55 G) UNSALTED BUTTER

½ CUP (120 ML) LACTOSE-FREE OR NONDAIRY MILK

Chicken Filling

2 TABLESPOONS (28 ML) OLIVE OIL, DIVIDED

4 BONELESS, SKINLESS CHICKEN THIGHS, CUT INTO 1-INCH (2.5 CM) PIECES

1 TEASPOON KOSHER SALT, DIVIDED

½ TEASPOON FRESHLY GROUND BLACK PEPPER, DIVIDED

½ CUP (50 G) SLICED SCALLIONS (GREEN PARTS ONLY)

1 STALK OF CELERY, THINLY SLICED

1 CUP (130 G) THINLY SLICED CARROTS

1½ CUPS (355 ML) UNSALTED CHICKEN STOCK OR CHICKEN BROTH (PAGE 109 OR 110)

1 TEASPOON POULTRY HERB SEASONING (PAGE 40)

½ CUP (120 ML) LACTOSE-FREE OR NONDAIRY MILK

2 TABLESPOONS (20 G) BASIC FLOUR BLEND (PAGE 38)

To prepare the biscuit dough, in a large bowl, whisk together the Basic Flour Blend, sugar, baking powder, and kosher salt. Cut in the butter until crumbly. Pour in the milk and mix until all of the flour is incorporated. Set aside.

To prepare the filling, preheat the oven to 400°F (200°C, or gas mark 6). In a large cast-iron or ovenproof skillet, heat 1 tablespoon (15 ml) of olive oil over medium-high heat. Season the chicken with ½ teaspoon each of the kosher salt and black pepper. Add the chicken and cook until browned and cooked through, about 6 to 8 minutes. Remove from the pan and set aside.

Reduce the heat to medium and add the remaining 1 tablespoon (15 ml) olive oil. Sauté the scallions and celery until slightly tender, about 4 to 5 minutes. Add the carrots and chicken stock. Simmer for about 15 minutes or until the carrots are tender.

Stir in the poultry herb seasoning and the remaining kosher salt and black pepper. In a small bowl, whisk together the milk and Basic Flour Blend. Slowly pour into the chicken stock or broth and vegetables in the skillet, while stirring constantly. Stir until thickened. Stir in the browned chicken.

Place dollops of biscuit dough evenly on top of the chicken filling. Place the skillet in the oven and bake for 15 to 17 minutes until the biscuit topping is lightly browned and the chicken filling is bubbling. Serve hot.

SWEDISH CHICKEN MEATBALLS

YIELD: 4 SERVINGS

My take on Swedish meatballs is another crowd-pleaser: Kids and adults will agree that these miniature meatballs are so much fun to eat. And you can make them both egg- and dairy-free, if you like: Just use a Chia Egg Replacer (see page 39), vegan margarine, and your favorite nondairy milk. Serve them over rice or gluten-free pasta if you like, so you can soak up every last drop of the savory sauce.

Meatballs

1 POUND (455 G) GROUND CHICKEN (90% LEAN)

½ CUP (51 G) QUINOA FLAKES, QUICK-COOKING OATS (40 G), OR BREAD CRUMBS (60 G) (PAGE 73)

½ CUP (50 G) SLICED SCALLIONS (GREEN PARTS ONLY)

1 LARGE EGG OR 1 CHIA EGG REPLACER (PAGE 39)

½ TEASPOON GROUND NUTMEG

½ TEASPOON KOSHER SALT

¼ TEASPOON FRESHLY GROUND BLACK PEPPER

1 TABLESPOON (15 ML) EXTRA-VIRGIN OLIVE OIL

Sauce

2 TABLESPOONS (28 G) UNSALTED BUTTER

½ CUP (50 G) SLICED SCALLIONS (GREEN PARTS ONLY)

¼ CUP (60 ML) LACTOSE-FREE OR NONDAIRY MILK

3 TABLESPOONS (30 G) BASIC FLOUR BLEND (PAGE 38)

3 TABLESPOONS (45 ML) DRY SHERRY OR DRY WHITE WINE

1 TEASPOON DIJON MUSTARD

2 CUPS (475 ML) CHICKEN BROTH OR CHICKEN STOCK (PAGE 110 OR 109)

¼ CUP (15 G) CHOPPED FRESH ITALIAN PARSLEY

½ TEASPOON KOSHER SALT

½ TEASPOON FRESHLY GROUND BLACK PEPPER

To make the meatballs, in the bowl of a stand mixer, blend together the ground chicken, quinoa flakes, scallions, egg, nutmeg, kosher salt, and black pepper. Roll into 1½-inch (4 cm) balls.

Heat the olive oil in a large skillet over medium-high heat. Add the meatballs and brown on all sides. Remove the meatballs from the skillet and set aside.

To make the sauce, melt the butter in the same skillet over medium heat. Add the scallions and cook until tender, about 1 to 2 minutes.

In a small bowl, stir together the milk, Basic Flour Blend, sherry or white wine, and Dijon mustard. Pour the mixture into the butter and scallions in the skillet and stir. Slowly pour in the chicken broth or stock while constantly stirring. Continue to stir until the sauce is thick and bubbly, about 5 minutes. Stir in the chopped fresh parsley and the kosher salt and black pepper.

Transfer the meatballs back to the skillet. Stir to coat the meatballs with the sauce. Continue to cook until the meatballs reach an internal temperature of 165°F (74°C). Serve hot.

TURKEY SHEPHERD'S PIE

YIELD: 4 SERVINGS

This updated, low-FODMAP version of the family-friendly classic is every bit as good as the original, and it's a bit lighter, too, since it uses lean ground turkey in place of beef. The herbed turkey mixture is topped with a blanket of garlicky potatoes and a few generous handfuls of cheese—and it's impossible to resist.

1¼ POUNDS (570 G) LEAN GROUND TURKEY

2 TABLESPOONS (28 G) UNSALTED BUTTER OR OLIVE OIL (28 ML)

¾ CUP (98 G) CHOPPED CARROTS

½ CUP (50 G) CHOPPED CELERY

½ CUP (50 G) SLICED SCALLIONS (GREEN PARTS ONLY)

3 TABLESPOONS (30 G) BASIC FLOUR BLEND (PAGE 38)

1½ CUPS (355 ML) CHICKEN BROTH OR CHICKEN STOCK (PAGE 110 OR 109)

1 TEASPOON POULTRY HERB SEASONING (PAGE 40)

1 TEASPOON KOSHER SALT

½ TEASPOON FRESHLY GROUND BLACK PEPPER

1 BATCH PARMESAN GARLIC SMASHED POTATOES (PAGE 88)

1 CUP (115 G) SHREDDED COLBY-JACK CHEESE

Preheat the oven to 350°F (180°C, or gas mark 4). Lightly grease a 2½-quart (2.4 L) casserole dish.

Crumble and brown the ground turkey in a large skillet over medium heat. Drain the fat and remove the turkey from skillet. Melt the butter in the same skillet. Add the carrots, celery, and scallions and sauté over medium heat until tender, about 7 to 8 minutes. Reduce the heat to low and sprinkle the vegetables with the Basic Flour Blend. Slowly whisk in the chicken broth or stock and stir until smooth. Cook until thick and bubbly, about 2 to 3 minutes. Stir in the cooked ground turkey and season with the poultry herb seasoning, kosher salt, and black pepper.

Spread the turkey mixture evenly in the prepared casserole dish. Spoon the smashed potatoes on top and spread them over the turkey in an even layer. Sprinkle with the shredded Colby-Jack cheese and bake for 20 to 25 minutes until the cheese is melted and the casserole is hot and bubbly. Serve immediately.

BROILED TURKEY TENDERS

YIELD: 4 SERVINGS

Turkey isn't just for deli sandwiches and Thanksgiving! This is a low-FODMAP adaptation of a recipe that my parents make all the time. (I'm not sure of its origins, but they've been making it forever.) Once you try it, you'll understand why. It's so simple to prepare that it hardly counts as cooking: You just mix a few basic ingredients into a marinade, pour it over the turkey, and then broil it a couple hours later. And the meat turns out full-flavored and tender every time. Turn these turkey tenders into a meal by adding a side of Baked Brown Rice with Parmesan and Herbs (page 97) and a small serving of steamed green beans. Or, chop them up and toss them into your favorite salad for extra protein.

3 OR 4 TURKEY TENDERS (ABOUT 1¼ POUNDS, OR 570 G), CUT IN HALF CROSSWISE

½ CUP (120 ML) DRY RED WINE

¼ CUP (60 ML) LIGHT-TASTING OLIVE OIL

3 TABLESPOONS (45 ML) GLUTEN-FREE SOY SAUCE OR TAMARI

Place the turkey tenders in a large resealable plastic bag. Combine the red wine, olive oil, and soy sauce in a small bowl and pour over the tenders in the bag. Seal and refrigerate for 2 hours.

Preheat the broiler. Place the tenders on a broiler pan. Discard the marinade. Broil for 4 to 5 minutes on each side until the turkey is cooked through.

TURKEY KEEMA WITH VEGGIES

YIELD: 4 SERVINGS

Keema is a seasoned ground meat dish that's popular in many parts of South Asia. While traditional recipes usually call for lamb, my version features lean ground turkey, fresh vegetables, and plenty of low-FODMAP spices. Add some steamed brown basmati rice for extra fiber, and you've got yourself a complete meal.

1 POUND (455 G) LEAN GROUND TURKEY

½ CUP (120 ML) WATER

½ TEASPOON KOSHER SALT

½ TEASPOON GROUND GINGER

½ TEASPOON GROUND CUMIN

½ TEASPOON GROUND CORIANDER

¼ TEASPOON GROUND CINNAMON

¼ TEASPOON GROUND TURMERIC

1 CUP (130 G) THINLY SLICED CARROTS

1 CUP (120 G) THINLY SLICED ZUCCHINI

2 CUPS (60 G) FRESH BABY SPINACH

2 SCALLIONS (GREEN PARTS ONLY), SLICED

COOKED BROWN BASMATI RICE, FOR SERVING

Crumble and brown the ground turkey in a large skillet over medium-high heat. Cook until the meat is no longer pink. Reduce the heat to medium and stir in the water, kosher salt, ginger, cumin, coriander (if using), cinnamon, and turmeric. Stir in the carrots and zucchini. Bring to a simmer, cover, and cook for 7 to 8 minutes until the vegetables are tender, stirring occasionally and adding more water if necessary.

Add the spinach, cover, and cook for about 2 more minutes or until the spinach is wilted. Stir in the sliced scallions and serve hot over rice.

RED WINE OVEN POT ROAST WITH THYME GRAVY

YIELD: 6 TO 8 SERVINGS

My husband is a big meat-and-potatoes guy (and so am I!), so this classic pot roast, in which red wine and thyme add subtle layers of flavor to the meat, is right up his alley. I've included directions for making gravy here, but the gravy is optional. Unless you ask my husband, that is: It's his favorite part of the meal!

1 BEEF CHUCK ROAST (3 TO 4 POUNDS, OR 1.4 TO 1.8 KG)

1½ TEASPOONS KOSHER SALT

½ TEASPOON FRESHLY GROUND BLACK PEPPER

2 TABLESPOONS (28 ML) OLIVE OIL

1 CLOVE OF GARLIC, PEELED AND SMASHED, BUT KEPT WHOLE

½ CUP (120 ML) DRY RED WINE

1 CUP (235 ML) BEEF STOCK (PAGE 111)

1 TEASPOON DRIED THYME

1 POUND (455 G) RED POTATOES, CUT INTO 1½-INCH (4 CM) PIECES

1 CUP (240 G) BABY CARROTS

2 STALKS OF CELERY, BIAS-CUT INTO 2-INCH (5 CM) PIECES

1 BUNCH OF SCALLIONS (GREEN PARTS ONLY), THINLY SLICED

2 TABLESPOONS (16 G) CORNSTARCH

¼ CUP (60 ML) WATER

Preheat the oven to 300°F (150°C, or gas mark 2). Season the roast with the kosher salt and black pepper.

In a Dutch oven, heat the olive oil over medium-high heat. Add the garlic and sauté until browned. Remove the garlic and discard. Add the roast and brown for 2 to 3 minutes per side. Remove from the heat and remove the roast from the pan. Drain the fat. Deglaze the pan with the red wine, scraping up any brown bits. Stir in the beef stock and thyme. Add the roast back to the pan. Cover and bake for about 2 hours, basting occasionally and turning the roast over halfway through.

Add the potatoes, carrots, celery, and scallions to the Dutch oven. Stir to coat with the liquid. Cover and bake for 1½ to 2 hours, stirring once, until the vegetables and roast are tender.

To make the gravy, transfer the roast and vegetables to a serving platter and cover. Pour the beef stock mixture from the pan into a large glass measuring cup or fat separator. Skim off the fat and discard. Pour the stock mixture back into the Dutch oven and heat over medium heat. Whisk together the cornstarch and water in a small bowl. Slowly pour the slurry into the stock mixture while constantly stirring. Continue to stir for a few minutes until the gravy is thick and bubbly. Serve alongside the roast and vegetables.

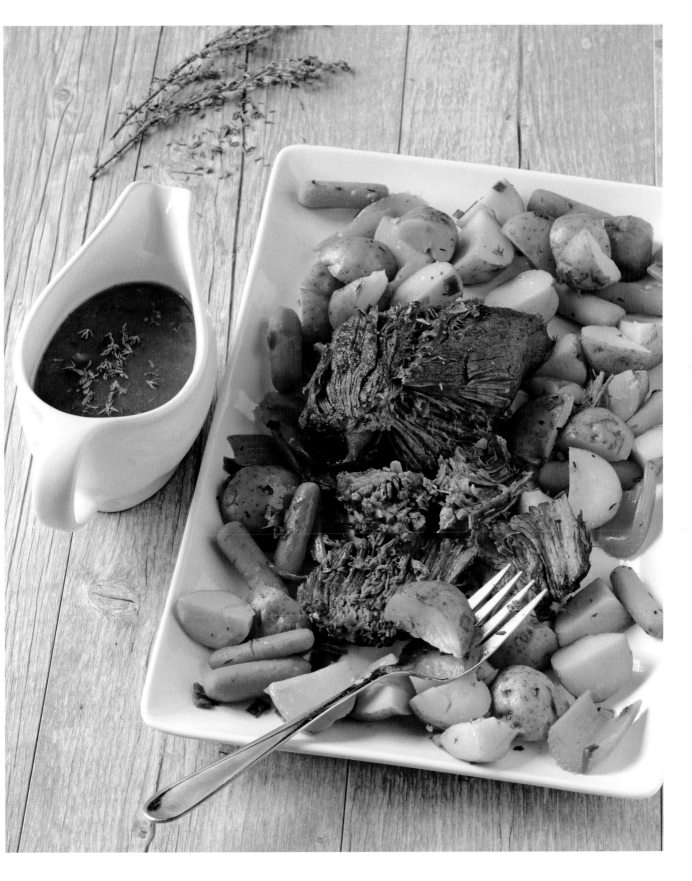

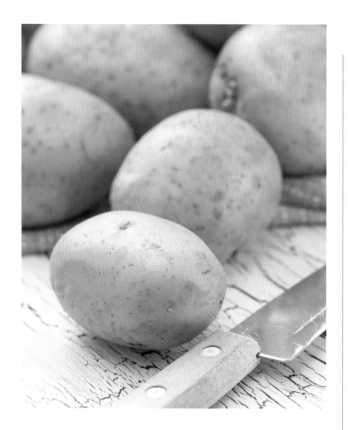

CHEESEBURGER AND FRIES CASSEROLE

YIELD: 4 SERVINGS

Think of this casserole as your favorite fast-food meal in a single dish—minus the processed, wheat-based bun and all the grease, of course! It was inspired by my mother-in-law's recipe for a Tater Tot hot dish, but to ensure that it's low-FODMAP, I whip up a quick béchamel-type sauce to use in place of condensed cream of mushroom soup. Be sure to check the ingredients list on the frozen French fries for FODMAPs. If you can't find any suitable fries, just make your own: Cut fresh potatoes into fry-size pieces and toss them with a little olive oil.

Casserole

1 POUND (455 G) GROUND BEEF

1 TABLESPOON (14 G) UNSALTED BUTTER OR MARGARINE

2 SCALLIONS (GREEN PARTS ONLY), SLICED

1 CUP (235 ML) BEEF STOCK, CHICKEN BROTH, OR VEGETABLE BROTH (PAGE 111, 110, OR 112)

½ CUP (120 ML) LACTOSE-FREE OR NONDAIRY MILK

3 TABLESPOONS (30 G) BASIC FLOUR BLEND (PAGE 38)

½ TEASPOON GROUND MUSTARD

¼ TEASPOON KOSHER SALT

¼ TEASPOON FRESHLY GROUND BLACK PEPPER

1 CUP (120 G) SHREDDED CHEDDAR CHEESE

1 PACKAGE (1 POUND, OR 455 G) CRINKLE-CUT FROZEN FRENCH FRIES

Preheat the oven to 425°F (220°C, or gas mark 7). Lightly grease a 2-quart (1.9 L) baking or casserole dish.

Brown the beef in a large skillet over medium-high heat until no longer pink. Transfer the cooked beef to a paper towel–lined plate to drain. Set aside.

Return the skillet to the heat and melt the butter over medium heat. Cook the scallions in the butter until tender, about 2 minutes. Add the stock or broth and bring to a simmer. In a small bowl or glass measuring cup, whisk together the milk and Basic Flour Blend. While constantly stirring, slowly pour the milk mixture into the skillet. Continue to cook and stir until thickened and bubbly. Stir in the ground mustard, kosher salt, and black pepper.

Ketchup

1 CUP (245 G) UNSALTED 100% TOMATO SAUCE

½ CUP (120 ML) RICE WINE VINEGAR

⅓ CUP (67 G) SUGAR

1 TEASPOON KOSHER SALT

Add the beef back to the skillet and stir into the sauce. Pour the mixture into the prepared baking dish and sprinkle evenly with the shredded cheddar cheese. Top with the frozen fries, spreading them out to cover the casserole. Bake for 25 to 30 minutes until the fries are golden brown.

Meanwhile, prepare the ketchup. Combine the tomato sauce, rice wine vinegar, sugar, and kosher salt in a medium saucepan and bring to a simmer. Simmer over low heat until thickened, about 20 minutes, stirring occasionally. Serve alongside, or drizzled on top of, the casserole.

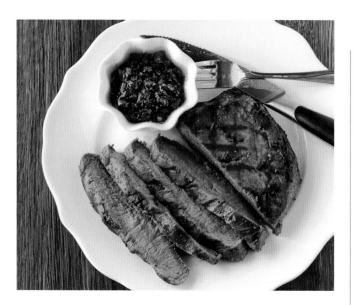

GRILLED FLAT IRON STEAK WITH CHIMICHURRI

YIELD: 4 SERVINGS

If you haven't tried flat iron steak before, now's the time. It's a shoulder cut, so it's more economical than popular cuts like rib eye, and but it's still tender and flavorful. And the low-FODMAP chimichurri sauce, made with parsley, cilantro, and garlic oil, is fabulous with grilled meat.

¾ CUP (175 ML) HOMEMADE GARLIC OLIVE OIL (PAGE 42)

3 TABLESPOONS (45 ML) RICE WINE VINEGAR, DIVIDED

1 TEASPOON KOSHER SALT, DIVIDED

1 TEASPOON FRESHLY GROUND BLACK PEPPER, DIVIDED

1 POUND (455 G) FLAT IRON STEAKS

1 CUP (60 G) PACKED FRESH ITALIAN PARSLEY

¼ CUP (4 G) FRESH CILANTRO LEAVES

1 TABLESPOON (4 G) FRESH OREGANO, OR 1 TEASPOON DRIED

Pour ¼ cup (60 ml) of the garlic oil into a large resealable plastic bag (refrigerate the remainder for later use in the chimichurri sauce). Add 2 tablespoons (28 ml) of the rice wine vinegar, ½ teaspoon of kosher salt, and ½ teaspoon of black pepper. Gently shake the bag to combine the ingredients. Add the steaks to the bag and shake to coat the meat. Marinate in the refrigerator for 2 to 4 hours.

Let the steaks come to room temperature (about 1 hour) before grilling. Prepare the chimichurri sauce by finely chopping the parsley and cilantro in a food processor. Transfer to a medium bowl and stir in the remaining ½ cup (120 ml) garlic oil, the remaining 1 tablespoon (15 ml) rice wine vinegar, the oregano, and the remaining ½ teaspoon kosher salt and ½ teaspoon black pepper.

Heat the grill to high. Grill the steak fillets for 4 to 5 minutes per side until they reach an internal temperature of 135°F (57°C) for medium-rare. Serve with the chimichurri sauce.

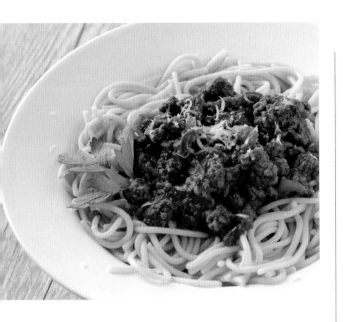

CLASSIC MEAT SAUCE FOR SPAGHETTI

YIELD: 6 SERVINGS

Since spaghetti with meat sauce was one of the first main dishes I learned to make as a kid, I just had to include a low-FODMAP version in this book. This recipe is all grown up, though: I've ramped up the herbs and added a splash of red wine for a meat sauce that's a bit more sophisticated than the one you loved when you were six. Serve it with brown rice spaghetti and a little grated Parmesan cheese.

1 POUND (455 G) LEAN GROUND BEEF

1 TABLESPOON (15 ML) OLIVE OIL

1 CLOVE OF GARLIC, PEELED AND SMASHED, BUT KEPT WHOLE

1 BUNCH OF SCALLIONS (GREEN PARTS ONLY), SLICED

¼ CUP (38 G) DICED GREEN BELL PEPPER

1 CUP (245 G) NO-SALT-ADDED 100% TOMATO SAUCE

1 CUP (180 G) NO-SALT-ADDED CANNED DICED TOMATOES, UNDRAINED

¼ CUP (60 ML) DRY RED WINE (OPTIONAL)

2 TEASPOONS DRIED BASIL

1 TEASPOON DRIED OREGANO

½ TEASPOON DRIED THYME

1 TEASPOON KOSHER SALT

½ TEASPOON FRESHLY GROUND BLACK PEPPER

1 BAY LEAF

Crumble and brown the beef in a large skillet over medium-high heat. Transfer the cooked beef to a paper towel–lined plate to drain.

Heat the olive oil in the skillet over medium heat. Add the garlic and cook until it starts to sizzle. Continue to cook for 1½ to 2 minutes more, just until the garlic starts to brown. Remove the garlic and discard it. Add the scallions and green bell pepper to the oil and sauté until tender, about 4 to 5 minutes. Add the beef back to the skillet. Stir in the tomato sauce, diced tomatoes, and red wine (if using). Stir in the basil, oregano, thyme, kosher salt, black pepper, and bay leaf.

Bring to a simmer and then reduce the heat to low. Simmer for 30 to 45 minutes until the sauce has thickened.

Remove the bay leaf and season to taste with kosher salt and black pepper, if desired.

HEARTY MEATLOAF

YIELD: 4 SERVINGS

Poor meatloaf. It tends to get a bad rap—for no good reason at all. Sure, it's plain, simple, and thrifty, but it's also filling and versatile. I've tried a few versions of meatloaf, and this is my best one yet: I can hardly believe it's low-FODMAP! Make it your own: For the binder, you can use quinoa flakes, oats, or bread crumbs, and if you're sensitive to eggs, use a Chia Egg Replacer (page 39) instead. Then, serve it with a homemade, ketchupy tomato sauce.

Sauce

½ CUP (123 G) NO-SALT-ADDED 100% TOMATO SAUCE

¼ CUP (60 ML) RICE WINE VINEGAR

3 TABLESPOONS (45 G) BROWN SUGAR

½ TEASPOON KOSHER SALT

Meatloaf

1½ POUNDS (680 G) LEAN GROUND BEEF

½ CUP (40 G) QUICK-COOKING OATS, QUINOA FLAKES (51 G), OR BREAD CRUMBS (60 G) (PAGE 73)

½ CUP (120 ML) LACTOSE-FREE OR NONDAIRY MILK

1 LARGE EGG OR 1 CHIA EGG REPLACER (PAGE 39)

½ CUP (50 G) SLICED SCALLIONS (GREEN PARTS ONLY)

1 TEASPOON KOSHER SALT

½ TEASPOON FRESHLY GROUND BLACK PEPPER

To make the sauce, combine the tomato sauce, rice wine vinegar, brown sugar, and kosher salt in a medium saucepan. Bring to a simmer and then reduce the heat to low and simmer, stirring occasionally, until thickened and reduced, about 20 minutes.

Meanwhile, preheat the oven to 350°F (180°C, or gas mark 4). Spray a 5 x 9-inch (13 x 23 cm) loaf pan with cooking spray.

Using a stand mixer, blend together the ground beef, oats, egg, scallions, kosher salt, and black pepper. Spread the meat mixture into the prepared pan. At this point, the sauce may be poured over top of the loaf or it can be set aside to serve alongside the meatloaf.

Bake for 1 hour to 1 hour and 15 minutes until the internal temperature reaches 160°F (71°C). Slice and serve hot.

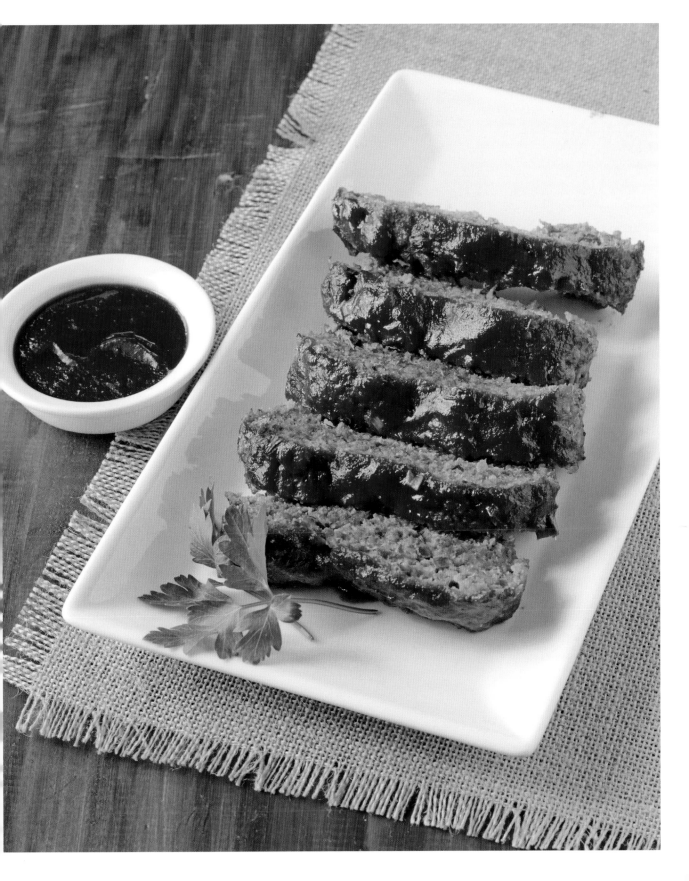

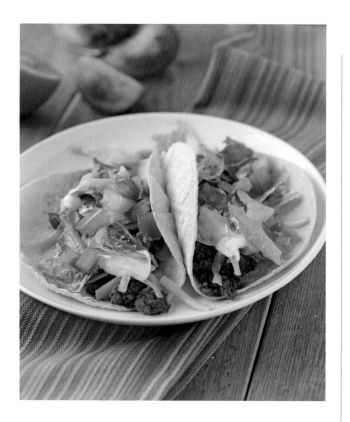

BEEF TACOS

YIELD: 4 SERVINGS

Who doesn't love tacos? Nobody in my house, anyway! This recipe may be low in FODMAPs—no garlic or onion necessary—but it's got plenty of punch. Just be sure to use pure ground chile powder rather than a chili powder blend: To get hold of it, you may need to consult with a clerk at your grocery store or health food store or shop online. (And be aware that ancho chile powder has not yet been tested for FODMAPs, so only use it if you know you can tolerate it.) Stuff the spiced taco meat and toppings into corn tortillas or other gluten-free alternatives: Food for Life makes a great brown rice tortilla, for instance. Or, skip the shells entirely and make a taco salad by serving the meat and toppings over a bed of lettuce.

1 POUND (455 G) GROUND BEEF

1½ TEASPOONS DRIED CHIVES

1 TEASPOON ANCHO CHILE POWDER (OPTIONAL)

1 TEASPOON CORNSTARCH

1 TEASPOON KOSHER SALT

¾ TEASPOON GROUND CUMIN

½ TEASPOON DRIED OREGANO

¼ TEASPOON FRESHLY GROUND BLACK PEPPER

¾ CUP (175 ML) WATER OR BEEF STOCK (PAGE 111)

CORN TORTILLA TACO SHELLS (HARD OR SOFT), FOR SERVING

SHREDDED CHEDDAR CHEESE, LACTOSE-FREE SOUR CREAM, SHREDDED LETTUCE, AND DICED TOMATOES, FOR SERVING

Brown the beef in a large skillet over a medium heat. Drain the excess fat. Stir in the chives, ancho chile powder, cornstarch, kosher salt, cumin, oregano, black pepper, and water or beef stock. Bring the mixture to a simmer and cook until thickened, about 10 minutes.

Serve the beef mixture in the taco shells and top with shredded cheddar cheese, sour cream, lettuce, and tomatoes.

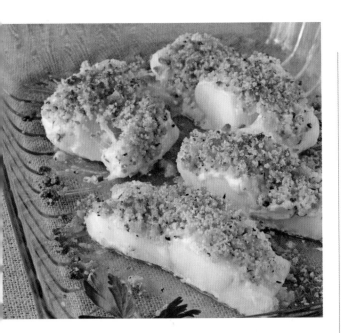

CRISPY BAKED COD

YIELD: 4 SERVINGS

Cod is, of course, fantastic when it's fried, but I prefer to bake it since the result is so much lower in fat. And, thanks to its mild, sweet taste, cod is a great backdrop for stronger flavors, like the home-made seasoned bread crumb mixture here. It's fast and easy enough to make on weeknights—even when you're working late—and it needs nothing more than a side of rice or quinoa and a salad, like the Citrus Fennel Carrot Slaw on page 80.

1 POUND (455 G) SKINLESS COD FILLETS

1 TABLESPOON (14 G) LIGHT MAYONNAISE

1 TEASPOON FRESH LEMON JUICE

⅓ CUP (38 G) BREAD CRUMBS (PAGE 73)

¼ CUP (25 G) GRATED PARMESAN CHEESE

1 TABLESPOON (15 ML) EXTRA-VIRGIN OLIVE OIL

1 TEASPOON ITALIAN HERB SEASONING (PAGE 40)

¼ TEASPOON KOSHER SALT

¼ TEASPOON FRESHLY GROUND BLACK PEPPER

Preheat the oven to 400°F (200°C, or gas mark 6). Lightly grease a 9 x 13-inch (23 x 33 cm) baking pan.

Place the cod fillets in the pan. In a small bowl, combine the mayonnaise and lemon juice. Spread evenly over each fillet.

In a medium bowl, combine the bread crumbs, Parmesan cheese, olive oil, Italian herb season-ing, kosher salt, and black pepper. Sprinkle the mixture evenly over the cod. Bake for 8 to 10 minutes until the topping is lightly browned and the cod easily flakes with a fork. Serve hot.

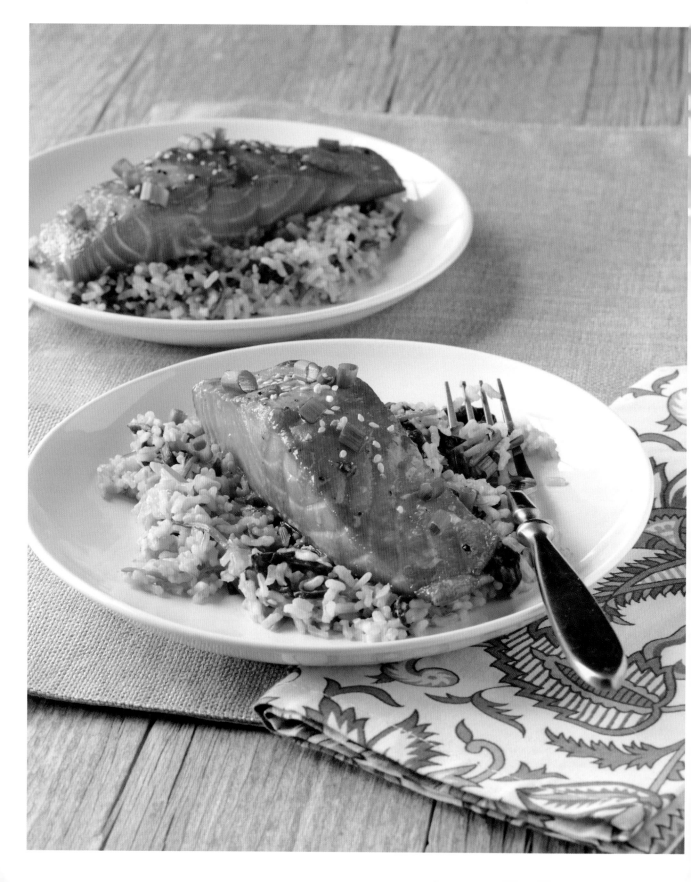

MAPLE-MARINATED SALMON WITH SESAME SPINACH RICE

YIELD: 4 SERVINGS

Oily fish like salmon is always a healthy choice, so you can feel good about serving this dish just about as often as you like. The maple-glazed salmon and sesame rice make a lovely sweet-and-savory combination, and the spinach provides a hefty dose of nutrients, like vitamin A and iron.

¼ CUP (60 ML) HOMEMADE GARLIC OLIVE OIL (PAGE 42)

¼ CUP (60 ML) PURE MAPLE SYRUP

2 TABLESPOONS (28 ML) GLUTEN-FREE SOY SAUCE OR TAMARI

¼ TEASPOON FRESHLY GROUND BLACK PEPPER

4 BONELESS, SKINLESS SALMON FILLETS (4 OUNCES, OR 115 G, EACH)

1¾ CUPS (425 ML) WATER

1 TEASPOON KOSHER SALT

2 CUPS (384 G) INSTANT BROWN RICE

1 TABLESPOON (8 G) RAW SESAME SEEDS

1 TABLESPOON (15 ML) TOASTED SESAME OIL

4 CUPS FRESH (120 G) BABY SPINACH

2 SCALLIONS (GREEN PARTS ONLY), SLICED

Put the garlic olive oil in a bowl and stir in the maple syrup, soy sauce, and black pepper. Place the salmon in a large resealable plastic bag. Pour in the maple syrup mixture and toss to coat the salmon. Refrigerate for about 4 hours to marinate.

Preheat the oven to 400°F (200°C, or gas mark 6). Line a baking sheet with aluminum foil and lightly coat with olive oil cooking spray. Place the salmon on the prepared baking sheet, drizzling a little of the marinade on top. Bake for 10 to 15 minutes until the salmon flakes with a fork.

Bring the water and kosher salt to a boil in a large saucepan. Stir in the rice and return to a boil. Reduce the heat to low and simmer, covered, for 5 minutes. Remove the rice from the heat and let it stand covered for another 5 minutes.

Heat a large dry skillet over medium heat. Add the sesame seeds and toast until lightly browned. Transfer the seeds to a small plate. In the same skillet, heat the sesame oil over medium heat. Add the spinach and sauté until wilted, about 2 to 3 minutes.

Stir the wilted spinach and toasted sesame seeds into the rice. Serve the salmon on top of the sesame spinach rice and sprinkle with the sliced scallions.

POTATO-CRUSTED TILAPIA WITH TANGY HERBED SAUCE

YIELD: 4 SERVINGS

Believe it or not, mashed potato flakes come in very handy if you're following a low-FODMAP eating plan—especially when it comes to "breading" fish. They lend the fish a delicate, crispy exterior that just begs for a zingy dipping sauce like this one, which sports fresh herbs, Dijon mustard, and seafood-friendly fresh lemon juice.

Tilapia

2 TABLESPOONS (20 G) RICE FLOUR

1 TEASPOON KOSHER SALT

¼ TEASPOON FRESHLY GROUND BLACK PEPPER

1 LARGE EGG, LIGHTLY BEATEN

½ CUP (26 G) MASHED POTATO FLAKES

1 POUND (455 G) TILAPIA FILLETS (OR OTHER WHITE FISH)

2 TABLESPOONS (28 ML) OLIVE OIL

2 TABLESPOONS (28 G) UNSALTED BUTTER

Tangy Herbed Sauce

½ CUP (115 G) LIGHT MAYONNAISE

1½ TABLESPOONS (25 ML) RICE WINE VINEGAR

1 TABLESPOON (3 G) MINCED FRESH CHIVES, OR 1 TEASPOON DRIED

1 TABLESPOON (4 G) MINCED FRESH ITALIAN PARSLEY, OR 1 TEASPOON DRIED

1 TEASPOON FRESH LEMON JUICE

½ TEASPOON DIJON MUSTARD

PINCH OF KOSHER SALT

PINCH OF FRESHLY GROUND BLACK PEPPER

To make the fish, combine the rice flour, kosher salt, and black pepper on a plate. Pour the lightly beaten egg onto another plate. Spread the potato flakes out on a third plate. Dip both sides of each tilapia fillet in the flour mixture, then the egg, and then the potato flakes.

Heat the olive oil and the butter together in a large skillet over medium-high heat. Brown the tilapia fillets for about 3 minutes per side or until the fish is browned and flakes easily with a fork.

To make the sauce, whisk together all of the ingredients in a small bowl until well blended. Serve alongside the fish fillets.

CREAMY PESTO TUNA PASTA

YIELD: 4 SERVINGS

This creamy pasta is another low-FODMAP adaptation of one of my childhood favorites, and it couldn't be easier to make. If you already have frozen portions of the broth and Spinach Basil Pesto on hand, it'll really come together in a flash. Add a side of steamed vegetables, and you've got a balanced weeknight meal.

3 CUPS (336 G) GLUTEN-FREE SPIRAL PASTA

¼ CUP (60 ML) LACTOSE-FREE OR NONDAIRY MILK

3 TABLESPOONS (30 G) BASIC FLOUR BLEND (PAGE 38)

1 CUP (235 ML) CHICKEN BROTH, CHICKEN STOCK, OR VEGETABLE BROTH (PAGE 110, 109, OR 112)

½ CUP (120 ML) SPINACH BASIL PESTO (PAGE 41)

2 CANS (5 OUNCES, OR 140 G EACH) LIGHT CHUNK TUNA IN WATER, DRAINED

¼ TEASPOON KOSHER SALT (OR TO TASTE)

¼ TEASPOON FRESHLY GROUND BLACK PEPPER (OR TO TASTE)

Bring a large pot of lightly salted water to a boil and cook the pasta according to the package directions. Drain and rinse with cold running water.

Combine the milk and Basic Flour Blend in a small bowl and stir until there are no lumps. In a large skillet, combine the broth or stock and Spinach Basil Pesto and bring to a simmer over medium-high heat. Reduce the heat to medium-low and, while constantly stirring, slowly pour the milk mixture into the skillet. Continue to cook and stir for a few minutes until thickened.

Add the tuna and cooked pasta and stir until well combined and heated. Season with the kosher salt and black pepper and serve.

ROASTED SALMON, POTATOES, AND BROCCOLI WITH ROSEMARY AND LEMON

YIELD: 4 SERVINGS

There are very few things that aren't better when they're roasted. And fish, vegetables, and potatoes are no exception to that rule—so why not pop them all into the oven on a single baking sheet for a quick, low-FODMAP dinner that requires minimal cleanup? I was delighted to find that broccoli is considered low-FODMAP in small servings—especially since roasting it gives it an addictively crispy, caramelized edge.

3 TABLESPOONS (45 ML) HOMEMADE GARLIC OLIVE OIL (PAGE 42)

1½ POUNDS (680 G) RED POTATOES, CUT INTO WEDGES

2 TEASPOONS CHOPPED FRESH ROSEMARY, DIVIDED

¾ TEASPOON KOSHER SALT, DIVIDED

¾ TEASPOON FRESHLY GROUND BLACK PEPPER, DIVIDED

2 CUPS (142 G) BROCCOLI FLORETS

1 POUND (455 G) WILD SALMON FILLET, PATTED DRY

1 TABLESPOON (15 ML) FRESH LEMON JUICE

Preheat the oven to 425°F (220°C, or gas mark 7). Line a large rimmed baking sheet with aluminum foil and spray with olive oil cooking spray.

In a large bowl, toss the potato wedges with 1 tablespoon (15 ml) of the garlic oil, 1 teaspoon of the rosemary, ¼ teaspoon of the kosher salt, and ¼ teaspoon of the black pepper. Spread the wedges out evenly on the prepared baking sheet and bake for 20 minutes.

While the potatoes are baking, toss together the broccoli, 1 tablespoon (15 ml) of the garlic oil, ¼ teaspoon of the kosher salt, and ¼ teaspoon of the black pepper in the same bowl you prepared the potatoes in.

Add the broccoli to the baking sheet with the browned potatoes. Push the potatoes and broccoli to the sides and place the salmon fillet in the middle of the sheet. Drizzle the salmon with the remaining 1 tablespoon (15 ml) garlic oil and sprinkle with the remaining 1 teaspoon rosemary, ¼ teaspoon kosher salt, and ¼ teaspoon black pepper.

Bake on the top rack of the oven for 10 to 15 minutes until the broccoli is browned and the salmon flakes easily. Drizzle with the lemon juice and serve.

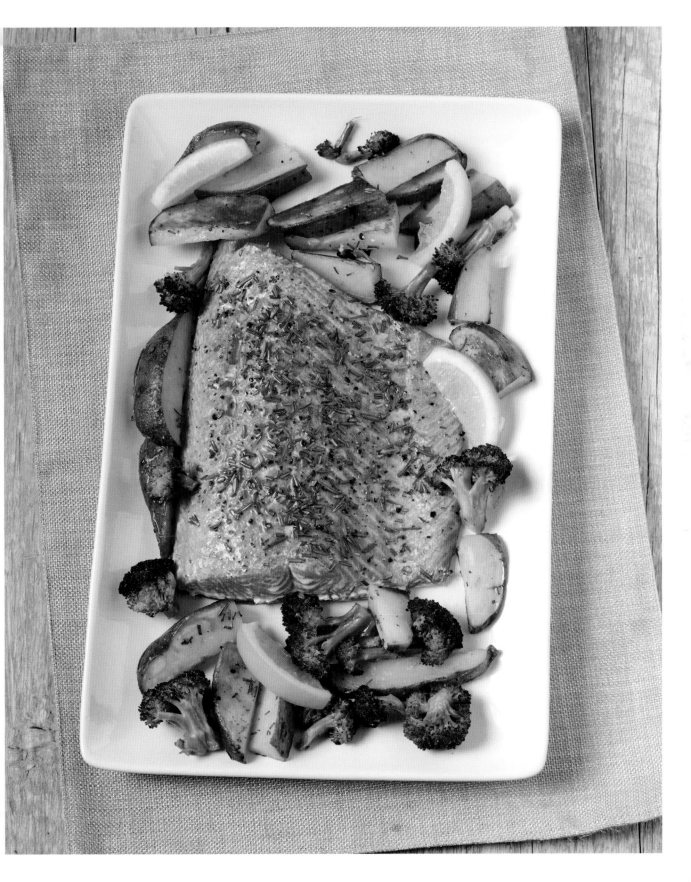

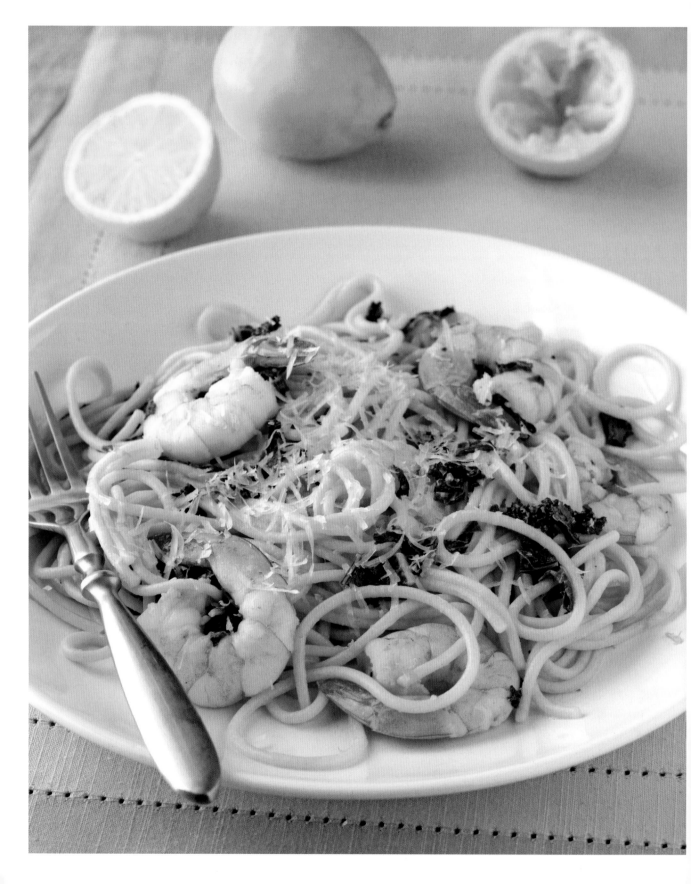

SHRIMP PASTA WITH LEMON AND KALE

YIELD: 4 SERVINGS

There's nothing difficult about this fresh, light, lemony pasta dish—it takes just minutes to make—but it's so elegant that you'll want to serve it the next time you have company over for dinner, or if you're planning a romantic night in. All it needs for an accompaniment is a crisp side salad.

8 OUNCES (225 G) RICE SPAGHETTI OR OTHER GLUTEN-FREE SPAGHETTI

2 TABLESPOONS (28 ML) OLIVE OIL

1 CLOVE OF GARLIC, PEELED

4 CUPS (268 G) CHOPPED FRESH KALE

1 POUND (455 G) SHRIMP, PEELED AND DEVEINED

½ TEASPOON GRATED LEMON ZEST

1 TABLESPOON (15 ML) FRESH LEMON JUICE

½ TEASPOON KOSHER SALT

½ TEASPOON FRESHLY GROUND BLACK PEPPER

¼ CUP (25 G) GRATED PARMESAN CHEESE (OPTIONAL)

Bring a large pot of lightly salted water to a boil and cook the spaghetti according to the package directions. Drain and rinse with cold running water.

Heat the olive oil in a large skillet over medium heat. Add the garlic and sauté for 1 to 2 minutes until the garlic starts to brown. Remove and discard the garlic.

Add the kale and shrimp to the skillet. Sauté until the kale is wilted and the shrimp is opaque, about 5 to 6 minutes.

Stir in the lemon zest, lemon juice, kosher salt, and black pepper. Add the spaghetti to the skillet and toss gently with a pair of tongs to combine and heat through. Serve sprinkled with the Parmesan cheese, if desired.

PORK CARNITAS WITH SLAW

YIELD: 8 OR MORE SERVINGS

Do you need a low-FODMAP recipe that can serve a crowd? Look no further. Shredded roast pork, or carnitas, makes great soft tacos. Your guests can top them with crunchy Lime Cabbage Slaw, or with traditional taco toppings like shredded cheese, lettuce, and tomatoes. Serve them with the Cilantro Lime Rice on page 100. (And if you're feeding a crowd, be sure to double the recipe for the slaw!)

Carnitas

2 TEASPOONS KOSHER SALT

2 TEASPOONS GROUND CUMIN

1 TEASPOON DRIED OREGANO

1 TEASPOON GROUND CORIANDER (OPTIONAL)

1 TEASPOON FRESHLY GROUND BLACK PEPPER

1 BAY LEAF

5 POUNDS (2.3 KG) BONELESS PORK SHOULDER ROAST, FAT TRIMMED

1 ORANGE, QUARTERED

1 BUNCH OF SCALLIONS (GREEN PARTS ONLY), CUT INTO 2-INCH (5 CM) PIECES

1 CUP (235 ML) CHICKEN STOCK, CHICKEN BROTH, VEGETABLE BROTH (PAGE 109, 110, OR 112), OR WATER

Lime Cabbage Slaw

½ CUP (115 G) LIGHT MAYONNAISE

1 TABLESPOON (15 ML) FRESH LIME JUICE

¼ TEASPOON EACH KOSHER SALT AND FRESHLY GROUND BLACK PEPPER

4 CUPS (280 G) SHREDDED CABBAGE-AND-CARROT BAGGED SLAW BLEND (AVOID SAVOY CABBAGE)

½ OF A BUNCH OF SCALLIONS (GREEN PARTS ONLY), SLICED

GLUTEN-FREE CORN TORTILLAS, WARMED ACCORDING TO PACKAGE DIRECTIONS, FOR SERVING

To make the carnitas, combine the kosher salt, cumin, oregano, coriander, and black pepper in a small bowl. Rub the mixture all over the pork roast. Place the pork roast in a large slow cooker, fat side up. Add the bay leaf and arrange the orange quarters and scallions around the roast. Carefully pour in the stock, broth, or water. Cook on the low setting for about 8 hours or on the high setting for about 4 hours.

Remove the roast from the slow cooker and use 2 forks to shred the meat. Place the shredded meat in a serving bowl. Remove bay leaf and and drizzle with the cooking liquid as needed to keep it moist.

To make the slaw, whisk together the mayonnaise, lime juice, kosher salt, and black pepper in a large bowl. Gently toss in the shredded cabbage and carrot blend and sliced scallions until well combined.

To serve, place the meat in warmed corn tortillas and top with the Lime Cabbage Slaw.

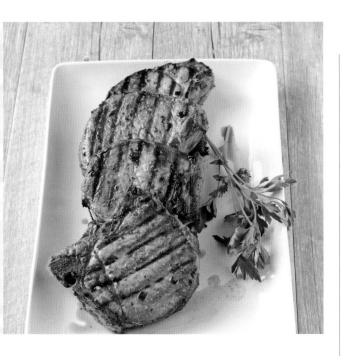

GRILLED MARINATED PORK CHOPS

YIELD: 4 SERVINGS

Oil, soy sauce, lemon juice—and maple syrup? That might sound like an unusual cast of characters, but together, they make an amazing marinade for pork chops (which works well with chicken, too). Serve them with Parmesan Garlic Smashed Potatoes (page 88) and Roasted Green Beans and Prosciutto (page 94). This recipe was inspired by a similar one on food.com.

⅓ CUP (80 ML) EXTRA-VIRGIN OLIVE OIL

⅓ CUP (80 ML) GLUTEN-FREE SOY SAUCE OR TAMARI

¼ CUP (60 ML) FRESH LEMON JUICE

2 TABLESPOONS (28 ML) PURE MAPLE SYRUP

4 SCALLIONS (GREEN PARTS ONLY), SLICED

1 TEASPOON DRIED OREGANO

½ TEASPOON FRESHLY GROUND BLACK PEPPER

4 THICK-CUT, BONE-IN PORK CHOPS

Combine the olive oil, soy sauce, lemon juice, maple syrup, scallions, oregano, and black pepper in a medium bowl. Place the pork chops in a large resealable plastic bag, pour the marinade over the pork chops, and seal the bag. Let the pork chops marinate in the refrigerator for 8 hours or up to overnight.

Heat the grill to medium heat and sear the pork chops on the grill, about 2 to 3 minutes per side. Move the chops away from direct heat and continue to cook until their internal temperature reaches 145°F (63°C), about 15 minutes. Serve immediately.

SLOW COOKER PORK CHOPS AND POTATOES

YIELD: 4 TO 6 SERVINGS

Recipes like this one, which features meat and potatoes in a creamy sauce, taste just like my childhood: pure comfort food. I've made a few changes, though: I use low-FODMAP chicken broth, and I've ditched the standard cream of mushroom soup in favor of my own homemade béchamel sauce. And I use a slow cooker, too; that way, I can get dinner taken care of hours in advance.

1 TABLESPOON (15 ML) OLIVE OIL

1 TO 1½ POUNDS (455 TO 680 G) BONELESS PORK CHOPS

2 TABLESPOONS (28 G) UNSALTED BUTTER OR MARGARINE

4 SCALLIONS (GREEN PARTS ONLY), SLICED

1 CUP (235 ML) CHICKEN BROTH, CHICKEN STOCK, OR VEGETABLE BROTH (PAGE 110, 109, OR 112)

½ CUP (120 ML) LACTOSE-FREE OR NONDAIRY MILK

3 TABLESPOONS (30 G) BASIC FLOUR BLEND (PAGE 38)

¼ CUP (60 ML) DRY WHITE WINE

2 TABLESPOONS (30 G) DIJON MUSTARD

¾ TEASPOON KOSHER SALT

½ TEASPOON FRESHLY GROUND BLACK PEPPER

½ TEASPOON DRIED BASIL

1½ POUNDS (680 G) POTATOES, CUT INTO ¼-INCH-THICK (6 MM) SLICES

Heat the olive oil in a large skillet over medium-high heat. Brown the pork chops in the oil, about 4 to 5 minutes on each side. Remove them from the skillet and set aside.

In the same skillet, reduce the heat to medium and melt the butter. Cook the scallions in the butter for about 30 seconds. Add the broth or stock and bring to a simmer. In a small bowl or glass measuring cup, combine the milk and Basic Flour Blend. While constantly stirring, slowly pour the milk mixture into the slkillet. Continue to cook and stir for a few minutes until thickened and bubbly. Stir in the white wine, Dijon mustard, kosher salt, black pepper, and basil.

Place the potatoes in the bottom of a large slow cooker. Pour half of the sauce over the potatoes. Place the browned pork chops on top and then top with the remaining sauce. Cook on the low setting for 8 hours or on the high setting for 4 hours. Serve hot.

PORK LO MEIN

YIELD: 4 SERVINGS

Luckily, it's often pretty easy to make Asian dishes low-FODMAP. (Just be sure to use regular green cabbage and avoid savoy cabbage, which is high in FODMAPs.) And don't be put off by what looks like a long list of ingredients; it's simple to make and comes together super fast. Feel free to use diced chicken breasts in place of the pork.

8 OUNCES (225 G) GLUTEN-FREE RICE SPAGHETTI

¼ CUP (60 ML) GLUTEN-FREE SOY SAUCE OR TAMARI

2 TABLESPOONS (28 ML) RICE WINE VINEGAR

4 TEASPOONS (11 G) CORNSTARCH

1 TEASPOON SUGAR

1 TEASPOON TOASTED SESAME OIL

½ TEASPOON GRATED FRESH GINGER

2 TABLESPOONS (28 ML) CANOLA OIL OR OTHER NEUTRAL OIL, DIVIDED

1 CLOVE OF GARLIC, PEELED AND SMASHED, BUT KEPT WHOLE

1 POUND (455 G) BONELESS PORK CHOPS, CUT INTO 1-INCH (2.5 CM) CUBES

¼ TEASPOON KOSHER SALT

¼ TEASPOON FRESHLY GROUND BLACK PEPPER

3 CUPS (210 G) SHREDDED GREEN CABBAGE

1 CUP (110 G) SHREDDED CARROTS

1 STALK OF CELERY, THINLY SLICED

1½ CUPS (355 ML) CHICKEN BROTH, CHICKEN STOCK, OR VEGETABLE BROTH (PAGE 110, 109, OR 112)

½ OF A BUNCH OF SCALLIONS (GREEN PARTS ONLY), SLICED

Bring a large pot of lightly salted water to a boil. Add the spaghetti and cook according to the package directions. Drain and rinse with cold water. Set aside.

In a small bowl, whisk together the soy sauce, rice wine vinegar, cornstarch, sugar, sesame oil, and ginger. Set aside.

Heat 1 tablespoon (15 ml) of the canola oil in large wok or skillet over medium-high heat. Add the garlic and sauté for 1 to 2 minutes, just until the garlic turns brown. Remove and discard the garlic.

Season the pork with the kosher salt and black pepper. Stir-fry for 4 to 5 minutes until browned and cooked through. Transfer to a plate and set aside.

In the same wok or skillet, heat the remaining 1 tablespoon (15 ml) canola oil over medium-high heat. Add the cabbage, carrots, and celery. Stir-fry until the vegetables are crisp-tender and are starting to brown, about 4 to 5 minutes.

Add the pork back to the wok. Stir in the broth or stock and the soy sauce mixture. Bring to a simmer and cook until the sauce is thickened. Toss in the spaghetti just to combine and reheat. Serve immediately, sprinkled with the sliced scallions.

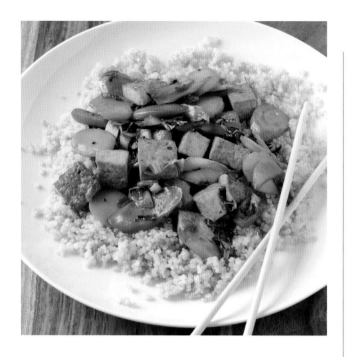

STIR-FRIED TOFU AND BOK CHOY

YIELD: 4 SERVINGS

I've learned that the trick to making tofu delicious is to sear it so that it's crisp and browned and to season it well with salt. (Tofu is as porous as a sponge, so it's important to drain it well before cooking; otherwise, it will be difficult to sear.) As for bok choy, it's very similar to Swiss chard: Its stems are edible, but they must be cooked for longer than the leaves. And both tofu and bok choy are delicious when they're bathed in a ginger-spiked, soy-based sauce like this one.

¼ CUP (60 ML) GLUTEN-FREE SOY SAUCE OR TAMARI

1 TABLESPOON (15 G) BROWN SUGAR

1 TABLESPOON (15 ML) RICE WINE VINEGAR

1 TABLESPOON (15 ML) TOASTED SESAME OIL

1 TEASPOON CORNSTARCH

½ TEASPOON MINCED FRESH GINGER

2 TABLESPOONS (28 ML) CANOLA OIL OR OTHER NEUTRAL OIL, DIVIDED

12 OUNCES (340 G) EXTRA-FIRM TOFU, DRAINED WELL AND CUT INTO CUBES

¼ TEASPOON KOSHER SALT

¼ TEASPOON FRESHLY GROUND BLACK PEPPER

2 CARROTS, THINLY BIAS-CUT

4 LARGE LEAVES OF BOK CHOY, STEMS THINLY BIAS-CUT, LEAVES CHOPPED

1 CAN (8 OUNCES, OR 225 G) SLICED WATER CHESTNUTS, DRAINED

4 SCALLIONS (GREEN PARTS ONLY), SLICED

COOKED RICE OR QUINOA, FOR SERVING

In a small bowl or glass measuring cup, whisk together the soy sauce, brown sugar, rice wine vinegar, sesame oil, cornstarch, and ginger. Set aside.

Heat 1 tablespoon (15 ml) of the canola oil in a large skillet over high heat. Add the tofu and cook until browned, about 2 to 3 minutes per side. Remove the tofu from the skillet and season with the kosher salt and black pepper.

Heat the remaining 1 tablespoon (15 ml) canola oil in the skillet over medium-high heat. Add the carrots and stir-fry for about 3 minutes. Add the bok choy stems and stir-fry until the carrots and stems are crisp-tender and lightly browned, about 3 minutes. Reduce the heat to low and carefully stir in the sauce mixture, tofu, bok choy leaves, water chestnuts, and scallions. Simmer for a few minutes until the sauce is thickened and the bok choy leaves are wilted. Serve over rice or quinoa.

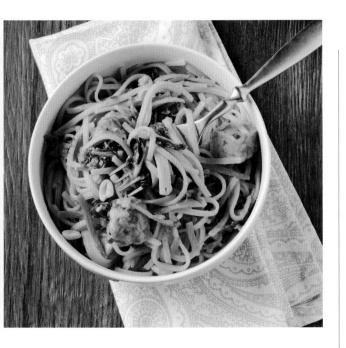

THAI PEANUT NOODLES WITH TEMPEH

YIELD: 4 SERVINGS

My husband took these noodles to work for lunch one day. He loved them—but he had no idea he was eating tempeh! He'd thought it was chicken, and, of course, I took that as a compliment. Share that story with anyone in your family who's uncertain about trying tempeh. It goes so well with these creamy, peanutty noodles. If you can tolerate it, pep them up with a pinch of red pepper flakes.

8 OUNCES (225 G) LINGUINE-STYLE STIR-FRY RICE NOODLES

¼ CUP (65 G) NATURAL CREAMY PEANUT BUTTER

3 TABLESPOONS (45 ML) GLUTEN-FREE SOY SAUCE OR TAMARI, DIVIDED

2 TABLESPOONS (28 ML) RICE WINE VINEGAR

1 TABLESPOON (15 ML) PURE MAPLE SYRUP

1 TABLESPOON (15 ML) TOASTED SESAME OIL

½ TEASPOON GRATED FRESH GINGER

1 TABLESPOON (15 ML) CANOLA OIL OR OTHER NEUTRAL OIL

1 CLOVE OF GARLIC, PEELED

8 OUNCES (225 G) TEMPEH, CUT INTO 1-INCH (2.5 CM) CUBES

1 CUP (110 G) SHREDDED CARROTS

4 CUPS (120 G) FRESH BABY SPINACH

½ OF A BUNCH OF SCALLIONS (GREEN PARTS ONLY), SLICED

½ CUP (8 G) CHOPPED FRESH CILANTRO

Bring a large pot of lightly salted water to a boil and cook the noodles according to the package directions. Reserve ¼ cup (60 ml) of the cooking liquid. Drain and rinse in cold running water. Set aside.

In a small bowl, combine the peanut butter, 2 tablespoons (28 ml) of the soy sauce, the rice wine vinegar, maple syrup, sesame oil, and ginger.

In a wok or large skillet, heat the canola oil over medium-high heat. Add the garlic and sauté until browned, about 1 to 2 minutes, and then remove the garlic from the pan and discard. Add the remaining 1 tablespoon (15 ml) soy sauce, the tempeh, and the carrots to the wok and stir-fry until the tempeh is lightly browned and the carrots are tender, about 5 minutes. Add the reserved cooking liquid from the noodles, the spinach, and the scallions. Stir-fry until the spinach is wilted, about 1 to 2 minutes.

Add the peanut sauce and noodles and toss gently to combine and heat through. Serve sprinkled with the chopped fresh cilantro.

PIZZA, THREE WAYS

YIELD: MAKES 1 PIZZA EACH (12 INCHES, OR 30 CM)

What's better than a recipe for pizza? Three recipes for pizza, that's what: a classic tomato-and-cheese version, a chicken pesto version, and a BLT pizza, in which spinach stands in for the lettuce and light mayonnaise takes the place of sauce. If you're having trouble deciding which one to try first, start by making my delicious traditional-style crust and then go from there.

Pizza Crust

2¼ TEASPOONS (ONE 0.25-OUNCE PACKET, OR 9 G) ACTIVE DRY YEAST

2 TABLESPOONS (26 G) SUGAR, DIVIDED

1 CUP (235 ML) WARM WATER (110°F, OR 43°C)

2½ CUPS (405 G) BASIC FLOUR BLEND (PAGE 38)

1 TEASPOON ITALIAN HERB BLEND (PAGE 40)

½ TEASPOON SALT

½ TEASPOON BAKING POWDER

1 TABLESPOON (15 ML) EXTRA-VIRGIN OLIVE OIL

Classic Tomato Pizza Sauce

1 CUP (245 G) NO-SALT-ADDED 100% TOMATO SAUCE

1 TABLESPOON (15 ML) HOMEMADE GARLIC OIL (PAGE 42)

2 TEASPOONS ITALIAN HERB BLEND (PAGE 40)

½ TEASPOON ANCHOVY PASTE (OPTIONAL) (CHECK PRODUCT INGREDIENTS FOR FODMAPS)

½ TEASPOON DRIED CHIVES

½ TEASPOON KOSHER SALT

¼ TEASPOON FRESHLY GROUND BLACK PEPPER

Preheat the oven to 425°F (220°C, or gas mark 7). Lightly grease a 12-inch (30 cm) pizza pan (no need to grease if you're using a nonstick pizza pan).

To make the pizza crust, in a medium bowl, combine the yeast and 1 tablespoon (13 g) of the sugar. Slowly pour in the warm water. Let the mixture sit for 5 to 10 minutes until it has formed a foamy head.

In a large bowl, combine the Basic Flour Blend, the remaining 1 tablespoon (13 g) sugar, the Italian herb blend, kosher salt, and baking powder. Add the olive oil and the yeast mixture. Stir well until there are no lumps. (The mixture will be more like a batter than a dough.)

Spread the mixture over the prepared pizza pan using a silicone spatula or greased hands. Par-bake the crust for 8 minutes; when done, the top of the crust will have a "crackled" appearance.

To make the Classic Tomato Pizza Sauce, combine all of the ingredients well in a small bowl.

Add desired toppings as follows and bake for 8 to 10 minutes more or until the pizza is hot and the cheese is melted and bubbly.

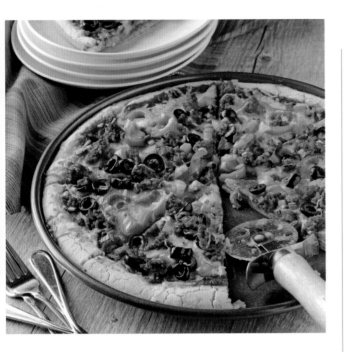

CHICKEN PESTO PIZZA

1 PIZZA CRUST (PAGE 164)

½ CUP (120 ML) SPINACH BASIL PESTO (PAGE 41)

1 CUP (140 G) SHREDDED COOKED CHICKEN BREAST

1 CUP (115 G) SHREDDED MOZZARELLA CHEESE

Prepare and par-bake the pizza crust according to the directions on page 164. Spread with the Spinach Basil Pesto Sauce and sprinkle evenly with the shredded chicken, followed by the shredded mozarella cheese. Finish baking according to the directions on page 164.

BLT PIZZA

1 PIZZA CRUST (PAGE 164)

½ CUP (115 G) LIGHT MAYONNAISE

1 TEASPOON DRIED BASIL

½ TEASPOON DRIED OREGANO

¼ TEASPOON FRESHLY GROUND BLACK PEPPER

2 ROMA TOMATOES, THINLY SLICED

½ POUND (225 G) BACON, COOKED CRISP, DRAINED, AND CRUMBLED (TRY TURKEY BACON FOR LESS FAT)

1 CUP (30 G) FRESH BABY SPINACH

1 CUP (115 G) SHREDDED MOZZARELLA CHEESE

Prepare and par-bake the pizza crust according to the directions on page 164. Spread with the mayonnaise and sprinkle with the basil, oregano, and black pepper. Cover evenly with the sliced tomatoes, bacon, and spinach. Sprinkle the shredded mozzarella cheese evenly on top. Finish baking according to the directions on page 164.

CLASSIC SUPREME PIZZA

1 PIZZA CRUST (PAGE 164)

1 BATCH CLASSIC TOMATO PIZZA SAUCE (PAGE 164)

¼ POUND (115 G) GROUND BEEF, CRUMBLED, BROWNED, AND DRAINED

½ CUP (75 G) CHOPPED GREEN OR RED BELL PEPPER OR A COMBO

1 CAN (2.25 OUNCES, OR 62 G) SLICED BLACK OLIVES, DRAINED

2 SCALLIONS (GREEN PARTS ONLY), SLICED

1 CUP (115 G) SHREDDED MOZZARELLA CHEESE

Prepare and par-bake the pizza crust according to the directions on page 164. Spread with the Classic Tomato Pizza Sauce and sprinkle evenly with the beef, bell pepper, black olives, scallions, and shredded mozzarella cheese. Finish baking according to the directions on page 164.

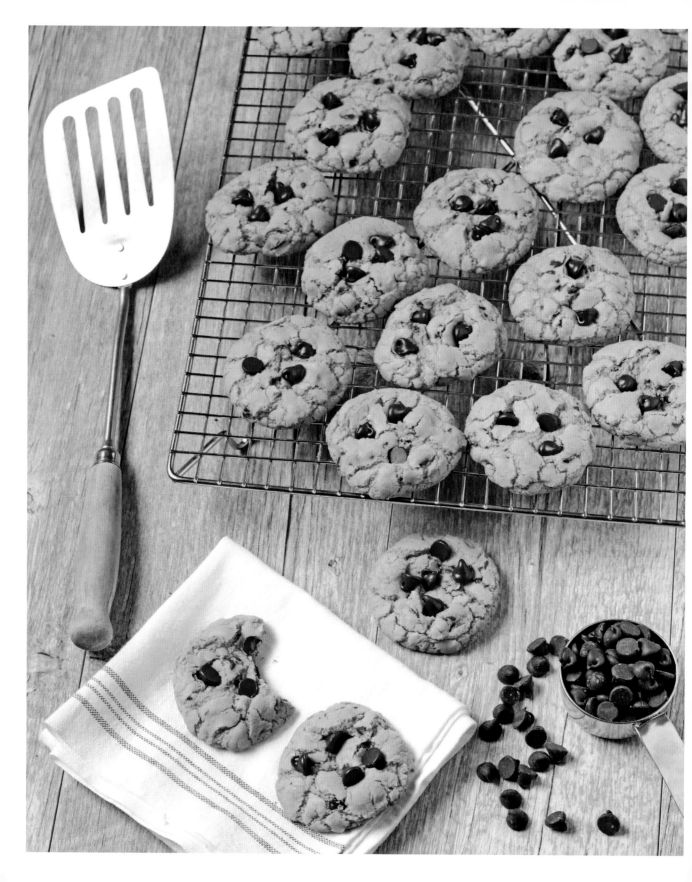

TREATS

8

You're on a low-FODMAP diet, but that doesn't mean you don't get to enjoy treats from time to time! Looking for a quick snack, a decadent dessert, or just something sweet to nibble with a cup of coffee? This chapter has got it all. You will learn how to make everything from homemade graham crackers to coconut-spiked lemon bars to chocolate chip cookies. I also show you to make some seriously impressive crowd-pleasing desserts, like a carrot cake that's drizzled with a brown butter glaze and a fruit galette that's much simpler to whip up than traditional fruit pies. If you're a chocoholic like me, you'll need to know what to do when you're faced with a major craving, and the answer is my One-Minute Vegan Chocolate Cake: It's got just a handful of ingredients, and it cooks in, yes, a minute.

What's more, all of the recipes in this chapter are wheat-free and aren't overloaded with sugar, which means they're easy to fit into your diet—whether you're in the elimination phase or you've already determined your tolerance levels. Many are vegan or vegan-adaptable, and all of them are so good that you'll want to share them with your friends and family. Best of all, no one will know that they're low-FODMAP—except you.

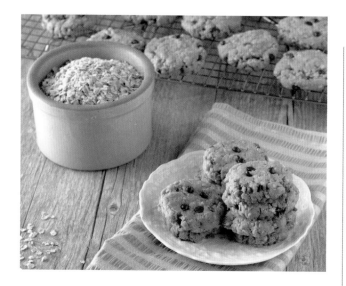

PEANUT BUTTER OATMEAL COOKIES

YIELD: 26 COOKIES

Inspired by "monster" cookies, which are loaded with peanut butter and chocolate (and just about everything else under the sun), these cookies are just as decadent. Use an easy-to-find brand of peanut butter that's free from molasses (and therefore low-FODMAP), like Skippy. While I love natural peanut butter and use it in lots of my recipes, it's a bit too thin to use in these cookies.

4 TABLESPOONS (55 G) UNSALTED BUTTER, SOFTENED

¾ CUP (195 G) CREAMY PEANUT BUTTER

½ CUP (100 G) GRANULATED SUGAR

¼ CUP (60 G) PACKED BROWN SUGAR

1 LARGE EGG OR 1 CHIA EGG REPLACER (PAGE 39)

1 TEASPOON PURE VANILLA EXTRACT

½ CUP (81 G) BASIC FLOUR BLEND (PAGE 38)

1 CUP (80 G) QUICK-COOKING OATS (GLUTEN-FREE IF NECESSARY)

½ TEASPOON BAKING SODA

¼ TEASPOON SALT

2 TABLESPOONS (22 G) FINELY CHOPPED DARK CHOCOLATE (OR MINI SEMISWEET CHOCOLATE CHIPS, IF TOLERATED)

Preheat the oven to 325°F (160°C, or gas mark 3). Line cookie sheets with parchment paper or lightly grease them.

Combine the butter, peanut butter, granulated sugar and brown sugar in the large bowl of a stand mixer. Beat on medium speed until creamy. Add the egg and vanilla and beat until combined. In a separate medium bowl, stir together the Basic Flour Blend, oats, baking soda, and salt. Add the flour mixture to the butter and sugar mixture and beat until combined. Stir in the chopped dark chocolate.

Form the dough into 1¼-inch (3 cm) balls and place them on the prepared cookie sheets. Flatten out the balls into approximately ½-inch-thick (1.3 cm) disks. Bake for 10 to 12 minutes until the cookies are just starting to brown lightly on the bottom edges. Let the cookies cool for at least 5 minutes on the cookie sheets before transferring them to a wire rack.

Make it vegan! Just use vegan margarine instead of butter and the Chia Egg Replacer in place of a real egg.

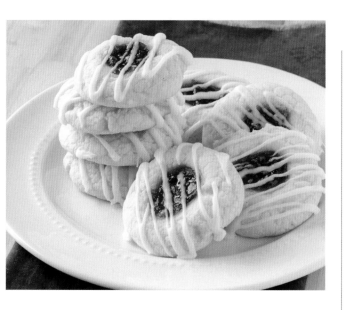

RASPBERRY THUMBPRINT COOKIES

YIELD: 24 COOKIES

These cookies are a holiday dessert-tray staple, but they're also great year-round. Just be sure to avoid excess fructose by using a jam that does not contain high-fructose corn syrup. Organic brands are usually trustworthy since most of them are made with pure sugar, not HFCS.

Cookies

6 TABLESPOONS (85 G) UNSALTED BUTTER, SOFTENED

¾ CUP (150 G) GRANULATED SUGAR

1 LARGE EGG

½ TEASPOON PURE ALMOND EXTRACT

½ TEASPOON SALT

2 CUPS (324 G) BASIC FLOUR BLEND (PAGE 38)

½ CUP (160 G) RASPBERRY JAM (CHECK PRODUCT INGREDIENTS FOR FODMAPS)

Glaze

1 CUP (120 G) CONFECTIONERS' SUGAR

2 TO 3 TEASPOONS (10 TO 15 ML) WATER

¼ TEASPOON PURE ALMOND EXTRACT

Preheat the oven to 375°F (190°C, or gas mark 5). Line cookie sheets with parchment paper or lightly grease them.

Cream the butter and sugar together in the large bowl of a stand mixer on medium speed until light and fluffy. Add the egg, almond extract, and kosher salt and beat until creamy. Turn the mixer to low; slowly add the Basic Flour Blend and beat until fully incorporated.

Roll the dough into 1¼-inch (3 cm) balls and place them on the prepared cookie sheets about 2 inches (5 cm) apart. Use your thumb to make an indentation on the top of each cookie. Fill each indentation with ¼ teaspoon of the jam.

Bake for 8 to 10 minutes until the bottom edges just start to lightly brown. Let the cookies cool for at least 5 minutes on the baking sheet before transferring them to a wire rack.

Prepare the glaze by mixing together the confectioners' sugar, water, and almond extract in a small bowl. Add more water by the half-teaspoonful, if necessary. Drizzle the glaze over the cooled cookies.

COCONUT SNICKERDOODLES

YIELD: 24 COOKIES

If you've never used coconut oil before, now's the time to give it a try. I started using it a couple of years ago and I really enjoy it—mostly for its subtle flavor. Although I'm more than a little skeptical about whether coconut oil really has the magical healing or fat-burning powers that some people claim it does, it sure is a good substitute for butter in vegan recipes, and it adds variety to your diet, too. Plus, it's delicious in these cookies, which are like a cross between the sophisticated coconut macaroon and that beloved childhood favorite, the snickerdoodle.

1¼ CUPS (200 G) BROWN RICE FLOUR

¼ CUP (20 G) UNSWEETENED FLAKED COCONUT

1 TEASPOON CREAM OF TARTAR

½ TEASPOON BAKING SODA

¼ TEASPOON SALT

½ CUP (100 G) PLUS 2 TABLESPOONS (26 G) GRANULATED SUGAR, DIVIDED

½ CUP (113 G) VIRGIN COCONUT OIL

1 LARGE EGG OR 1 CHIA EGG REPLACER (PAGE 39)

1 TEASPOON PURE VANILLA EXTRACT

½ TEASPOON GROUND CINNAMON

Preheat the oven to 375°F (190°C, or gas mark 5). Line cookie sheets with parchment paper.

In a medium bowl, stir together the rice flour, coconut, cream of tartar, baking soda, and salt.

In the large bowl of a stand mixer, beat the ½ cup (100 g) sugar and the coconut oil on medium speed until light and fluffy, about 2 minutes. Blend in the egg and vanilla. Add the flour mixture and mix until thoroughly combined.

Stir the 2 tablespoons (26 g) sugar and cinnamon together in a small bowl. Roll the dough into 1½-inch (4 cm) balls. Roll each ball in the cinnamon sugar mixture and place on the prepared cookie sheets. Flatten each ball slightly using the back of a spoon.

Bake for 10 to 11 minutes until lightly golden. Let the cookies cool for at least 5 minutes on the baking sheet before transferring them to a wire rack.

Make it vegan! Simply use the Chia Egg Replacer (page 39) instead of a regular egg.

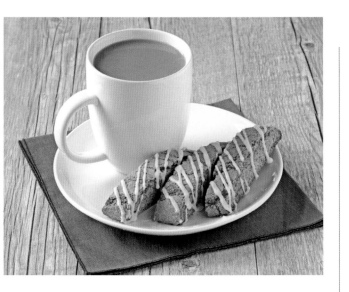

GINGERBREAD BISCOTTI

YIELD: ABOUT 16 COOKIES

My festive, low-FODMAP take on classic Italian biscotti turns out cookies that are light, crisp, and perfect for dunking into all sorts of hot beverages.

Preheat the oven to 325°F (160°C, or gas mark 3). Line a large cookie sheet with parchment paper.

In a medium bowl, whisk together the Basic Flour Blend, chia seeds, baking powder, ginger, cinnamon, nutmeg, salt, and ground cloves.

In the large bowl of a stand mixer, beat the egg until frothy. Add the brown sugar and beat until glossy. Turn the mixer to low and slowly add the flour mixture. Continue to mix until the flour is well incorporated; the dough will be soft and slightly sticky.

Shape the dough into a round log about 8 inches (20 cm) long, flattening the top of the log slightly. Bake for about 30 minutes or until the top is firm to the touch and lightly browned.

Remove the log from the oven and let it cool on a wire rack for 15 minutes. Then slice it diagonally into ½-inch (1.3 cm) slices. Carefully turn each slice over onto its side and place it cut side down on the cookie sheet. Return to the oven and bake the slices for 8 minutes. Turn each slice over onto the other cut side and bake for another 6 to 8 minutes until lightly browned. Let the biscotti cool for at least 5 minutes on the baking sheet before transferring them to the wire rack.

To make the glaze, combine the confectioners' sugar and water. Drizzle over the cooled biscotti.

Biscotti

1¼ CUPS (203 G) BASIC FLOUR BLEND (PAGE 38)

2 TEASPOONS GROUND CHIA SEEDS

1 TEASPOON BAKING POWDER

1 TEASPOON GROUND GINGER

½ TEASPOON GROUND CINNAMON

¼ TEASPOON GROUND NUTMEG

¼ TEASPOON SALT

⅛ TEASPOON GROUND CLOVES

1 LARGE EGG

½ CUP (115 G) PACKED DARK BROWN SUGAR

Glaze

½ CUP (60 G) CONFECTIONERS' SUGAR

2 TEASPOONS WATER

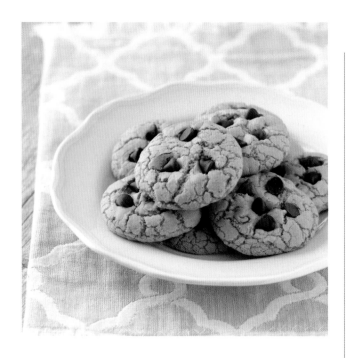

CHOCOLATE CHIP COOKIES

YIELD: 24 COOKIES

I've worked magic with these cookies, if I do say so myself: They're low-FODMAP and reduced fat! And they're crispy on the outside but chewy inside—the ideal combination, in my opinion. Chocolate chips have not been tested, so stick with the chopped dark chocolate during the strict phase of the diet. To make your cookies picture-perfect, set aside some of the chopped chocolate and press a few onto the top of each cookie right after they come out of the oven.

2 CUPS (324 G) BASIC FLOUR BLEND (PAGE 38)

½ TEASPOON SALT

½ TEASPOON BAKING SODA

½ TEASPOON BAKING POWDER

4 TABLESPOONS (55 G) UNSALTED BUTTER, SOFTENED, OR VIRGIN COCONUT OIL (56 G)

½ CUP (115 G) PACKED BROWN SUGAR

¼ CUP (50 G) GRANULATED SUGAR

1 LARGE EGG OR 1 CHIA EGG REPLACER (PAGE 39)

1 TEASPOON PURE VANILLA EXTRACT

1 CUP (175 G) CHOPPED DARK CHOCOLATE (OR SEMISWEET CHOCOLATE CHIPS, IF TOLERATED), DIVIDED

Preheat the oven to 375°F (190°C, or gas mark 5). Line cookie sheets with parchment paper.

Stir together the Basic Flour Blend, salt, baking soda, and baking powder in a large bowl. In the large bowl of a stand mixer, beat the softened butter, brown sugar, and granulated sugar until creamy. Beat in the egg and vanilla. Add the flour mixture and mix until well blended. Stir in ⅔ cup (117 g) of the chopped dark chocolate (reserving ⅓ cup [58 g] to press onto the tops of the cookies).

Roll the dough into 1½-inch (4 cm) balls and place on the prepared cookie sheets, 12 per sheet. Do not flatten. Bake, one sheet at a time, for 8 to 10 minutes until the bottoms of the cookies are just barely beginning to turn golden. As soon as you remove the cookies from the oven, press 4 or 5 pieces of chocolate onto the top of each cookie. Let the cookies cool for at least 5 minutes on the baking sheet before transferring them to a wire rack.

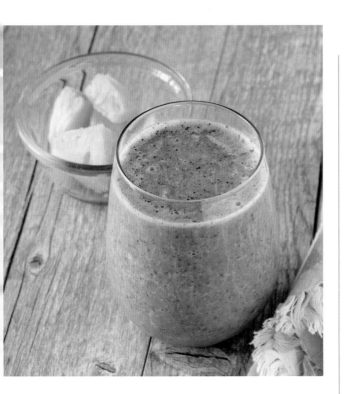

BANANA SMOOTHIES, THREE WAYS

YIELD: 1 SERVING EACH

When you're craving something that's sweet but a bit healthier than a cookie or a slice of cake, make one of these delicious smoothies. Try freezing bananas for your smoothies when they're just ripe enough: Simply lay sliced banana pieces out on a baking sheet and transfer to the freezer. When the banana slices are frozen, store them in the freezer in a resealable plastic bag and use them as you need them. And to make any of these smoothies even more filling, just add a scoop of rice protein powder.

PB & J SMOOTHIE

1 CUP (235 ML) LACTOSE-FREE OR NONDAIRY MILK

½ OF A RIPE BANANA, SLICED AND FROZEN

5 FROZEN STRAWBERRIES

1 TABLESPOON (16 G) NATURAL CREAMY PEANUT BUTTER (OR 2 TABLESPOONS [12 G] POWDERED PEANUT BUTTER)

1 TEASPOON PURE MAPLE SYRUP

CHOCOLATE PEANUT BUTTER SMOOTHIE

¾ CUP (175 ML) LACTOSE-FREE OR NONDAIRY MILK

½ OF A RIPE BANANA, SLICED AND FROZEN

1 TABLESPOON (16 G) NATURAL CREAMY PEANUT BUTTER (OR 2 TABLESPOONS [12 G] POWDERED PEANUT BUTTER)

1½ TEASPOONS UNSWEETENED COCOA POWDER

1 TEASPOON PURE MAPLE SYRUP

PINEAPPLE GREEN SMOOTHIE

1 CUP (235 ML) LACTOSE-FREE OR NONDAIRY MILK

1 CUP (30 G) FRESH BABY SPINACH

½ OF A RIPE BANANA, SLICED AND FROZEN

½ CUP (85 G) FROZEN PINEAPPLE CHUNKS

1 TEASPOON PURE MAPLE SYRUP

To make each smoothie, simply combine all of the ingredients in a blender and blend until smooth. Serve immediately.

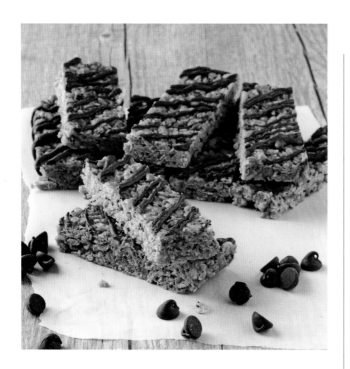

CHEWY PEANUT BUTTER GRANOLA BARS

YIELD: 10 BARS

Chocolate and peanut butter are absolutely irresistible, just like these granola bars. My granola bars are made with light corn syrup, which is composed mostly of glucose—so, while it hasn't yet been tested for FODMAPs, most light corn syrups like Karo shouldn't cause problems for a low-FODMAP diet. (Be careful with generic brands, though, since many of them do contain high-fructose corn syrup.)

Granola Bars

1 CUP (80 G) QUICK-COOKING OATS
(GLUTEN-FREE IF NECESSARY)

¾ CUP (23 G) GLUTEN-FREE CRISPY BROWN
RICE CEREAL

¼ CUP (36 G) ROASTED SUNFLOWER SEEDS

1 TABLESPOON (13 G) CHIA SEEDS

⅓ CUP (80 ML) LIGHT CORN SYRUP

¼ CUP (65 G) NATURAL PEANUT BUTTER

3 TABLESPOONS (39 G) SUGAR

½ TEASPOON PURE VANILLA EXTRACT

Chocolate Drizzle

⅓ CUP (58 G) CHOPPED DARK CHOCOLATE

1 TEASPOON NATURAL PEANUT BUTTER

Line an 8-inch (20 cm) square baking pan with aluminum foil and spray with cooking spray.

In a large bowl, combine the oats, rice cereal, sunflower seeds, and chia seeds.

In a small, microwave-safe bowl, stir together the corn syrup, peanut butter, sugar, and vanilla. Microwave on high for 60 seconds. Stir.

Drizzle the peanut butter mixture over the rice cereal mixture and stir until well combined. Transfer to the prepared pan and press down on the mixture firmly with the back of a clean spoon or lightly greased hands to spread it out evenly. Let cool.

To make the topping, melt the chocolate and peanut butter in a microwave-safe bowl on high for 30 seconds. Stir until smooth. Microwave for an additional 15 seconds if needed. Drizzle the topping over the cooled bars.

Let the chocolate harden and cut it into bars to serve.

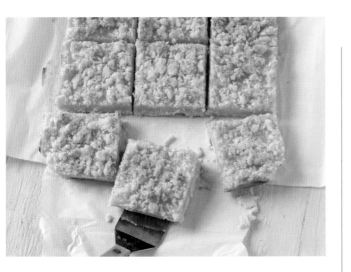

COCONUT LEMON BARS

YIELD: 16 BARS

Coconut gussies up the zesty lemon in these sweet-and-tart dessert bars. They've got a crust that's made with virgin coconut oil, and they're dressed up with a topping of toasted flaked coconut.

1½ CUPS (243 G) BASIC FLOUR BLEND (PAGE 38)

½ CUP (60 G) CONFECTIONERS' SUGAR

1 TEASPOON GRATED LEMON ZEST

¼ TEASPOON SALT

½ CUP (113 G) VIRGIN COCONUT OIL

¼ CUP (20 G) UNSWEETENED FLAKED COCONUT

¼ CUP (60 ML) PLUS 1 TO 2 TEASPOONS WATER, DIVIDED

¾ CUP (150 G) GRANULATED SUGAR

2 TABLESPOONS (16 G) CORNSTARCH

2 LARGE EGGS

1 LARGE EGG YOLK

3 TABLESPOONS (45 ML) FRESH LEMON JUICE

Preheat the oven to 400°F (200°C, or gas mark 6). Line an 8-inch (20 cm) square baking pan with parchment paper.

Stir together the Basic Flour Blend, confectioners' sugar, lemon zest, and salt. Cut in the coconut oil until crumbly. Put ⅓ cup (85 g) of this mixture into a small bowl and stir in the coconut flakes. Set this aside for the topping.

To the remaining coconut oil mixture, add the water, a teaspoon at a time, working the dough with your hands until the mixture starts to come together. Press into the bottom of the pan and bake for 14 to 16 minutes until the crust starts to brown.

In a large saucepan, combine the granulated sugar and cornstarch. In a medium bowl, whisk the eggs and egg yolk well. Stir in the ¼ cup (60 ml) water and the lemon juice. Pour this mixture into the saucepan with the sugar and cornstarch. Cook, while constantly stirring, over medium heat just until thickened and bubbly, about 10 minutes. Pour the mixture over the baked crust and sprinkle evenly with the reserved topping mixture. Bake for 13 to 15 minutes until the coconut is lightly toasted. Cool completely before cutting into bars.

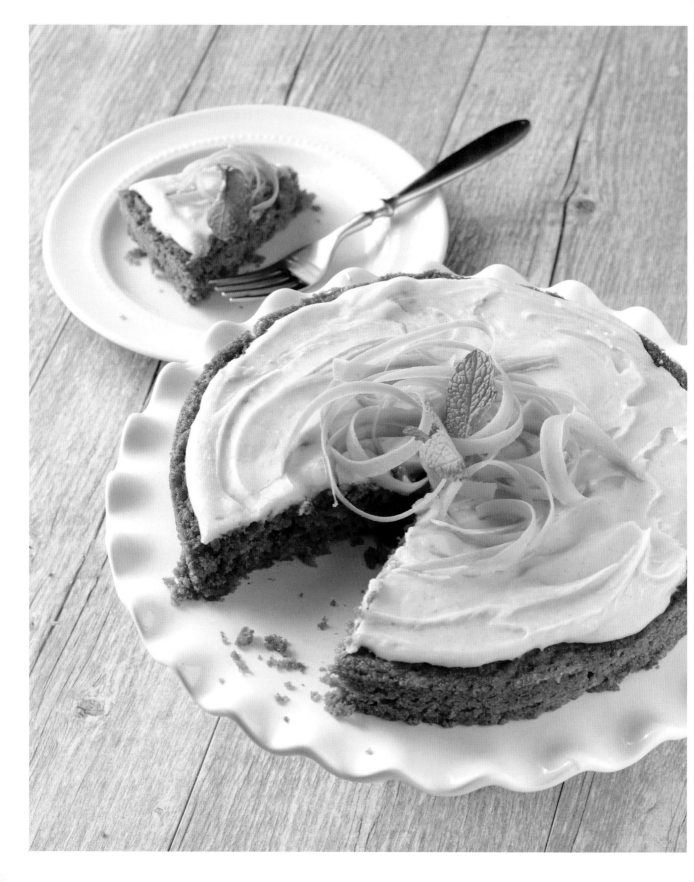

CARROT CAKE WITH BROWNED BUTTER GLAZE

YIELD: 12 SERVINGS

Carrot cake is my favorite cake in the whole world, and I make it every year to celebrate my husband's and my wedding anniversary. Since cream cheese is high in lactose, this low-FODMAP version skips the standard cream cheese–laden frosting in favor of a rich, vanilla-tinged brown butter glaze that isn't overwhelmingly sweet. It's the perfect complement to the spiced cake.

Cake

1¼ CUPS (203 G) BASIC FLOUR BLEND (PAGE 38)

1 TEASPOON GROUND CINNAMON

½ TEASPOON BAKING POWDER

½ TEASPOON BAKING SODA

¼ TEASPOON SALT

¼ TEASPOON GROUND NUTMEG

2 LARGE EGGS

½ CUP (100 G) GRANULATED SUGAR

¼ CUP (60 G) PACKED BROWN SUGAR

⅓ CUP (80 ML) CANOLA OIL OR OTHER NEUTRAL OIL

2 CUPS (220 G) SHREDDED CARROTS

Glaze

3 TABLESPOONS (42 G) UNSALTED BUTTER

1 TABLESPOON (15 ML) LACTOSE-FREE MILK, PLUS MORE IF NEEDED

½ TEASPOON PURE VANILLA EXTRACT

1 CUP (120 G) CONFECTIONERS' SUGAR

Preheat the oven to 350°F (180°C, or gas mark 4). Line a 9-inch (23 cm) round cake pan with parchment paper and spray the sides with cooking spray.

To make the cake, in a medium bowl, stir together the Basic Flour Blend, cinnamon, baking powder, baking soda, salt, and nutmeg. In a large bowl, beat the eggs, granulated sugar, brown sugar, and canola oil. Beat in the shredded carrots. Add the flour mixture and blend well. Pour the batter into the prepared cake pan. Bake for 30 to 35 minutes until a toothpick comes out clean. Let the cake cool completely on a wire rack before turning it out onto a serving platter.

To make the glaze, melt the butter in a medium saucepan over low heat. Continue to cook until the butter is lightly browned, about 3 to 4 minutes. Stir in the milk and vanilla. Add the confectioners' sugar and stir until smooth. Add more milk, a teaspoon at a time, until the mixture reaches a pouring consistency. Pour over the plated cake and spread the glaze out using a spatula.

STRAWBERRY RHUBARB GALETTE WITH LEMONY WHIPPED CREAM

YIELD: 6 TO 8 SERVINGS

Rhubarb and strawberries are a natural match—and, luckily, they're both low-FODMAP, so I just had to combine the two in a pastry. Galettes are much easier to make than pies; they look pretty and rustic, and the crust doesn't have to be perfect. The citrusy whipped cream completes this wonderful warm-weather dessert.

Crust

1½ CUPS (243 G) BASIC FLOUR BLEND (PAGE 38)

2 TABLESPOONS (26 G) GRANULATED SUGAR, PLUS MORE FOR SPRINKLING

½ TEASPOON SALT

½ TEASPOON GRATED LEMON ZEST

6 TABLESPOONS (85 G) UNSALTED BUTTER, CUT INTO PIECES

2 TO 3 TABLESPOONS (28 TO 45 ML) WATER

Filling

2 CUPS (340 G) HULLED AND HALVED STRAWBERRIES

1 CUP (122 G) CHOPPED RHUBARB

¼ CUP (50 G) GRANULATED SUGAR

2 TABLESPOONS (20 G) BASIC FLOUR BLEND (PAGE 38)

LACTOSE-FREE MILK, FOR BRUSHING ON CRUST

Lemony Whipped Cream

1 CUP (235 ML) HEAVY WHIPPING CREAM

2 TABLESPOONS (28 ML) FRESH LEMON JUICE

¼ CUP (30 G) CONFECTIONERS' SUGAR

Preheat the oven to 425°F (220°C, or gas mark 7). Line a large cookie sheet with parchment paper.

To prepare the crust, place the Basic Flour Blend, sugar, salt, and lemon zest in a food processor or blender and pulse until combined. Add the butter and pulse again until the mixture resembles coarse meal. Add the water, a teaspoon at a time, pulsing after each addition, just until the dough starts to come together. Remove the dough from the food processor and form it into a disk. Place the dough onto the prepared baking sheet. Lightly flour the dough and roll out evenly into a 12-inch (30 cm) round. Set aside.

To make the filling, in a large bowl, toss the strawberries and rhubarb together with the sugar and the Basic Flour Blend. Mound the strawberry mixture in the middle of the crust, leaving about 2 inches (5 cm) of crust exposed at the edges. Use the parchment paper to help you fold the crust over the berry mixture, leaving the center exposed. Brush the crust with milk and sprinkle with the remaining sugar. Bake for 20 minutes or until the crust is golden brown and the fruit is bubbly. Let cool on a wire rack and cut into slices.

To make the Lemony Whipped Cream, beat the heavy cream until foamy. Add the lemon juice and confectioners' sugar and beat until stiff peaks form. Top each slice of the galette with the Lemony Whipped Cream and serve.

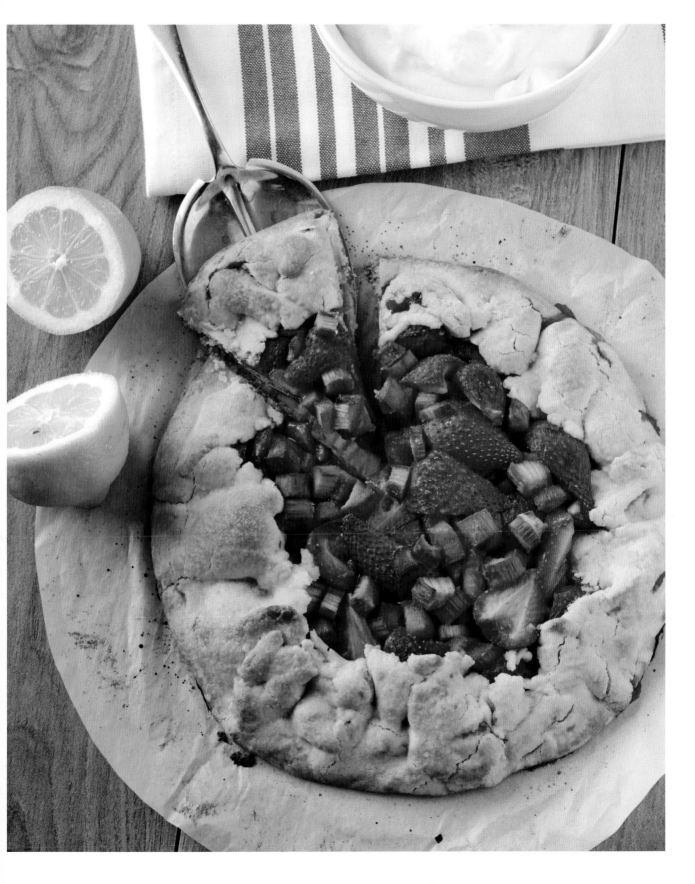

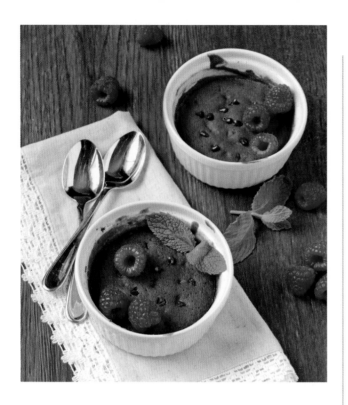

ONE-MINUTE VEGAN CHOCOLATE CAKE

YIELD: 1 SERVING

You know those late-night chocolate cravings that are impossible to shake once they strike? This microwave cake is the answer, so go ahead and indulge. (Okay, so this recipe does involve 90 seconds of microwaving time, plus dirtying up a bunch of measuring spoons—but trust me, you won't regret it!) For an extra-special treat, top it with a small scoop of low-FODMAP, lactose-free vanilla ice cream.

1½ TEASPOONS VIRGIN COCONUT OIL

1½ TEASPOONS LACTOSE-FREE OR NONDAIRY MILK

1 TABLESPOON (15 ML) PURE MAPLE SYRUP

¼ TEASPOON PURE VANILLA EXTRACT

2 TABLESPOONS (20 G) BASIC FLOUR BLEND
(PAGE 38)

1½ TEASPOONS UNSWEETENED COCOA POWDER

⅛ TEASPOON BAKING POWDER

PINCH OF SALT

1 TEASPOON FINELY CHOPPED DARK CHOCOLATE
(OR MINI SEMISWEET CHOCOLATE CHIPS, IF
TOLERATED)

Place the coconut oil in a microwave-safe bowl, mug, or ramekin. Microwave on high for about 30 seconds to melt the coconut oil.

Stir in the milk, maple syrup, and vanilla. Add the Basic Flour Blend, cocoa powder, baking powder, and salt and stir well. Stir in the chopped dark chocolate. Microwave on high for 1 minute and then serve immediately. (It's best eaten standing at the kitchen counter in your pajamas.)

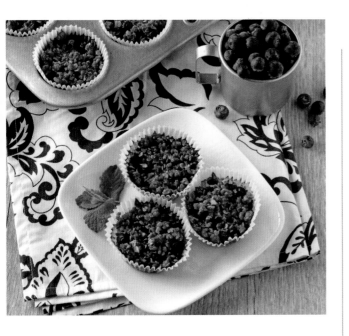

MINI BLUEBERRY CRISPS

YIELD: 6 SERVINGS

To tell you the truth, I'm not that great at baking fruit pies. But fruit crisps? I sure am good at those—all you need to do is dump everything into a dish and stick it in the oven! Blueberry crisp is one of my favorites, but if you're on a low-FODMAP diet, it's important to be mindful of serving sizes, as blueberries contain fructans. But with these individual mini crisps, it's easy to control both FODMAPs and calories at the same time.

3 TABLESPOONS (42 G) UNSALTED BUTTER OR VIRGIN COCONUT OIL

½ CUP (40 G) QUICK-COOKING OATS (GLUTEN-FREE IF NECESSARY)

⅓ CUP (75 G) PACKED BROWN SUGAR

¼ CUP (41 G) BASIC FLOUR BLEND (PAGE 38)

½ TEASPOON GROUND CINNAMON

¼ TEASPOON SALT

1 CUP (145 G) FRESH OR FROZEN BLUEBERRIES

Preheat the oven to 350°F (180°C, or gas mark 4). Double-line 6 cups of a standard-size muffin pan with paper liners.

Melt the butter in a medium saucepan over low heat. Remove the pan from the heat and stir in the oats, brown sugar, Basic Flour Blend, cinnamon, and salt. Stir until well combined and crumbly.

Press a heaping tablespoon (15 g) of the crisp mixture into the bottom of each muffin cup. Add about 20 blueberries to each cup. Sprinkle each cup evenly with the remaining crisp mixture. Bake for 30 to 35 minutes until the blueberries are bubbling and the tops are lightly browned. Serve warm.

Make it vegan! Use the coconut oil instead of the butter.

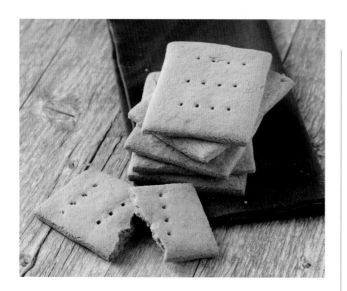

GRAHAM-STYLE CRACKERS

YIELD: ABOUT 20 CRACKERS

You'd think that graham crackers would be out of the question on a low-FODMAP eating plan. After all, graham is a type of wheat flour, and that means, unfortunately, that it's not a low-FODMAP food. Luckily, I came up with a recipe that comes pretty close to the traditional graham crackers you've loved since kindergarten.

2 CUPS (324 G) BASIC FLOUR BLEND (PAGE 38)

⅓ CUP (75 G) PACKED BROWN SUGAR

1 TEASPOON BAKING POWDER

1 TEASPOON GROUND CINNAMON

½ TEASPOON SALT

¼ TEASPOON BAKING SODA

4 TABLESPOONS (55 G) UNSALTED BUTTER OR VEGAN MARGARINE, CHILLED

¼ CUP (60 ML) PURE MAPLE SYRUP

1 TEASPOON PURE VANILLA EXTRACT

1 TABLESPOON (15 ML) WATER, PLUS MORE IF NEEDED

Preheat the oven to 325°F (160°C, or gas mark 3). Line a large cookie sheet with parchment paper.

In a large bowl, combine the Basic Flour Blend, brown sugar, baking powder, cinnamon, salt, and baking soda. Using a pastry blender or fork, cut in the butter until crumbly.

In a small bowl, combine the maple syrup, vanilla, and water. Add to the flour mixture. Using your hands, work the mixture until it comes together in a soft, pliable dough. Add more water, a teaspoon at a time, if needed, to make a pliable dough.

Roll the dough out on a well-floured surface (using the flour blend) or between sheets of parchment paper to a ⅛-inch (3 mm) thickness. Cut into 2 x 3-inch (5 x 7.5 cm) rectangles and transfer to the prepared cookie sheet, placing each rectangle ½ inch (1.2 cm) apart. Prick with a fork, if desired.

Bake for 26 to 28 minutes until the edges turn golden brown. Let the crackers cool for 1 to 2 minutes on the cookie sheet before transferring them to a wire rack.

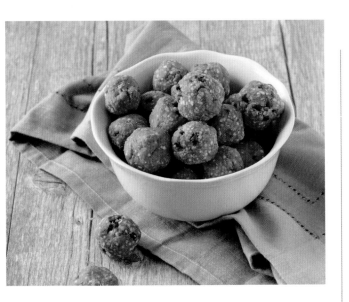

POWER POPPERS

YIELD: 18 TO 20 POPPERS

I love to keep a batch of these little nuggets in the fridge so that I can reach for one anytime I need a quick energy boost—like when I'm absolutely starving, but it's too close to dinnertime to make a full-on snack (which, somehow, seems to happen nearly every day). Packed with natural peanut butter, oats, coconut, and chocolate, they're so filling that just one is enough to tide you over until your next meal.

¾ CUP (195 G) NATURAL CREAMY PEANUT BUTTER

2 TABLESPOONS (28 ML) PURE MAPLE SYRUP

1 TEASPOON PURE VANILLA EXTRACT

½ TEASPOON GROUND CINNAMON

½ CUP (51 G) QUINOA FLAKES OR QUICK-COOKING OATS (40 G) (GLUTEN-FREE IF NECESSARY)

¼ CUP (20 G) UNSWEETENED SHREDDED COCONUT

2 TABLESPOONS (22 G) FINELY CHOPPED DARK CHOCOLATE (OR MINI SEMISWEET CHOCOLATE CHIPS, IF TOLERATED)

In a medium bowl, combine the peanut butter, maple syrup, vanilla, and cinnamon. Stir until smooth. Stir in the quinoa flakes, coconut, and the chopped dark chocolate. The mixture will be very thick; you may need to use your hands to combine the ingredients.

Roll the mixture into 1¼-inch (3 cm) balls. Refrigerate until firm. Store in the refrigerator for up to 2 weeks.

FASTENOWS' CRANBERRY CRUSH

YIELD: 16 SERVINGS

I'm so excited to share this old family recipe with you! My family serves this slushy frozen treat at Thanksgiving and Christmas instead of cranberry sauce, and as kids, we thought it was the best part of the holiday meal. Don't wait till the holidays to try it, though: Like sorbets, it also makes a refreshing summertime treat since frozen cranberries are usually available year-round. While dried cranberries and cranberry juice have been tested for FODMAPs, fresh cranberries have not, so this recipe may not be appropriate during the strict phase of the diet. Consult with your dietitian.

3 CUPS (700 ML) WATER

1 BAG (12 OUNCES, OR 340 G) FRESH OR FROZEN CRANBERRIES, RINSED AND DRAINED

2 CUPS (400 G) SUGAR

½ CUP (120 ML) FRESH ORANGE JUICE

1 TABLESPOON (15 ML) FRESH LEMON JUICE

Bring the water to a boil in a large pot. Add the cranberries and sugar. Lower the heat and gently boil for 10 minutes, stirring occasionally.

Place a coarse-mesh sieve over a freezer-safe 9 x 13-inch (23 x 33 cm) pan. Pour the cranberry mixture through the sieve, letting the juice drain into the pan. Use a wooden spoon to press down on the cranberries in order to extract all of the juice. Discard the cranberries or reserve them for another use.

Stir the orange and lemon juices into the cranberry juice in the pan and freeze overnight. Cut the crush into squares and serve in bowls. Slurp up every last drop with a spoon!

OVEN-ROASTED PEPITAS, TWO WAYS

YIELD: ABOUT 8 SERVINGS EACH

Pepitas are hulled pumpkin seeds, and they're an excellent source of protein, so they're a good choice if you're looking for a healthy snack that's not terribly sweet. Pepitas are especially delicious when they're oven-roasted, then treated to a thorough coating in cocoa powder or spices. Look for pepitas at your local health food store or shop online. (Be sure to watch your serving size, though, since pumpkin seeds do contain fructans.)

COCOA-ROASTED PEPITAS

1 CUP (160 G) RAW PEPITAS

2 TEASPOONS SUGAR

2 TEASPOONS UNSWEETENED COCOA POWDER

PINCH OF SALT

1 TABLESPOON (15 ML) WATER

½ TEASPOON PURE VANILLA EXTRACT

Preheat the oven to 300°F (150°C, or gas mark 2). Line a large rimmed baking sheet with parchment paper. Spread the pepitas out on the baking sheet and bake for 30 minutes.

Meanwhile, mix together the sugar, cocoa powder, and salt in a small bowl. Stir in the water and vanilla. After removing the pepitas from the oven, drizzle them with the chocolate mixture. Toss to evenly coat. Return to the oven for another 10 to 15 minutes until the pepitas are dry and crispy.

SPICE-ROASTED PEPITAS

1 CUP (160 G) RAW PEPITAS

1 TABLESPOON (15 G) BROWN SUGAR

1 TEASPOON GROUND CINNAMON

¼ TEASPOON GROUND GINGER

⅛ TEASPOON GROUND NUTMEG

PINCH OF GROUND CLOVES

PINCH OF SALT

1 TABLESPOON (15 ML) WATER

Preheat the oven to 300°F (150°C, or gas mark 2). Line a large rimmed baking sheet with parchment paper. Spread the pepitas out on the baking sheet and bake for 30 minutes.

Meanwhile, mix together the brown sugar, cinnamon, ginger, nutmeg, ground cloves, and salt in a small bowl. Stir in the water. After removing the pepitas from the oven, drizzle them with the spice mixture. Toss to evenly coat. Return to the oven for another 10 to 15 minutes until the pepitas are dry and crispy.

ACKNOWLEDGMENTS

This was a challenging but rewarding book to write, and there are some important people who helped me along the way.

Thank you to Jill Alexander, Heather Godin, Megan Buckley, and Renae Haines for giving me the opportunity to fulfill my dream of writing a cookbook and for all of your hard work in helping to shape this book into something I'm truly proud of.

Thank you to my husband, Bryan, for doing the vacuuming and laundry and being my shoulder to cry on. I truly couldn't have done this without you and I love you. Thanks to my parents for showing me the love of food and for always believing in me. Thanks to my dad for encouraging my interest in photography and to my mom for teaching me to cook and collect recipes. Thank you to my sister,

Andrea, for reminding me how capable I am. Thank you to my friend Missy for being my cheerleader.

A huge thanks to all of the family, friends, and co-workers who helped taste-test everything and relieve us of the constant buildup of cookies and muffins!

A special thank you to Jane Muir, Jane Varney, Maria Stevenberg, and Marina Iacovou with Monash University for consulting with me. Thank you to the rest of the Monash University team for the work and research you are doing. The app is so useful. Thank you to Patsy Catsos for the wonderful advice and to Kate Scarlata for your website and willingness to share about FODMAPs. And thanks to you both for bringing the low-FODMAP diet to the United States. There are a lot of happy bellies out there because of you.

ABOUT THE AUTHOR

Dianne Fastenow Benjamin transformed her love of cooking, baking, and photography into a food blog called Delicious as it Looks, where she loves to share her kitchen creations. After having so much success following a low-FODMAP diet to treat her IBS, she devotes most of her blog to Low-FODMAP foods and recipes.

Dianne works as a civil engineer in Cedar Rapids, Iowa, where she lives with her husband, Bryan, and two pugs, Stanley and Maggie. When she's not working, in the kitchen, or behind a camera, she enjoys reading, staying fit, and avoiding unloading the dishwasher.

SOURCES

Abo, B., Bevan J., Greenway, S., Healy, B., McCurdy, S., Peutz, J., Wittman, G. (2014 Oct). Making Garlic- and Herb-Infused Oils At Home. Retrieved from http://extension.uidaho.edu/owyhee/files/2013/10/PNW664-Making-Garlic-and-Herb-Infused-Oils-at-Home.pdf

Akbar, A., Yiangou, Y., Facer, P., Walters, J.R.F., Anand, P., Ghosh, S. (2008). Increased capsaicin receptor TRPV1-expressing sensory fibres in irritable bowel syndrome and their correlation with abdominal pain. *Gut.* 2008 Jul; 57 (7): 923-9.

Biesiekierski, J.R., Peters, S.L., Newnham, E.D., Rosella, O., Muir, J.G., Gibson, P.R. (2013 Aug). No Effects of Gluten in Patients with Self-Reported Non-Celiac Gluten Sensitivity After Dietary Reduction of Fermentable, Poorly Absorbed, Short-Chain Carbohydrates. *Gastroenterology.* 2013 Aug; 145(2): 320-8.

Brostoff, Jonathan, M.D. & Gamlin, Linda. (2000). *Food Allergies and Food Intolerance: The Complete Guide to Their Indentification and Treatment.* Rochester, VT: Healing Arts Press.

Brown, Alton. (2015 Mar). The Difference Between Stocks and Broths. Retrieved fromwww.altonbrown.com/the-difference-between-stocks-and-broths.

Catsos, Patsy, MS, RD, LD. (2012). *IBS Free at Last! Change Your Carbs, Change Your Life, with the FODMAP Elimination Diet* (2nd ed.). Portland, ME: Pond Cove Press.

Catsos, Patsy, MS, RD, LD. (2015 Apr). FODMAPs and Other Conditions. Retrieved from www.ibsfree.net/fodmaps-and-other-conditions

Catsos, Patsy, MS, RD, LD. (2014 May). FODMAPs and Soy: Why so Confusing? Retrieved from www.ibsfree.net/news/2014/5/18/fodmaps-and-soy-why-so-confusing

Code of Federal Regulations Title 21. (2014 Apr). 21CFR101.22 Foods; labeling of spices, flavorings, colorings, and chemical preservatives.

Cook's Country. (2014 Dec/Jan). Getting to Know: Umami Powerhouses. Retrieved from www.cookscountry.com/how_tos/8173-getting-to-know-umami-powerhouses

Dai, C., Zheng, C., Jiang, M., Ma, X., Jiang, L. (2013 Sep). Probiotics and irritable bowel syndrome. *World Journal of Gastroenterology* 2013 Sep; 19 (36): 5973-80

Duyff, Roberta Larson, MS, RD, FADA, CFCS. (2012). *American Dietetic Association Complete Food and Nutrition Guide.* Hoboken, NJ: John Wiley & Sons, Inc.

Scarlata, Kate, RD, LDN. (2014). *Low-FODMAP 28-Day Plan: A Healthy Cookbook with Gut-Friendly Recipes for IBS Relief.* Berkeley, CA: Rockridge Press.

Scarlata, Kate, RD, LDN. (2010). *The Complete Idiot's Guide to Eating Well with IBS.* New York, NY: Penguin Group.

Scarlata, Kate, RD, LDN. (2010, Aug). The FODMAPs Approach: Minimize Consumption of Fermentable Carbs to Manage Functional Gut Disorder Symptoms. *Today's Dietitian*, 12 (8), 30.

Scarlata, Kate, RD, LDN. (2012, Mar). Successful Low-FODMAP Living—Experts Discuss Meal-Planning Strategies to Help IBS Clients Better Control GI Distress. *Today's Dietitian*, 14 (3), 36.

Scarlata, Kate, RD, LDN. (2015 July). Low FODMAPs Grocery List. Retrieved from blog.katescarlata.com/fodmaps-basics/low-fodmap-shopping-list

Science Daily. (2015 Feb). Widely used food additives promotes colitis, obesity and metabolic syndrome, shows study of emulsifiers. Retrieved from www.sciencedaily.com/releases/2015/02/150225132105.htm

Shepherd, Sue, PhD & Gibson, Peter, MD. (2013). *The Complete Low-FODMAP Diet: A Revolutionary Plan for Managing IBS and Other Digestive Disorders*. New York: The Experiment Publishing.

The Monash University Low FODMAP App for smartphones. Apr 16, 2015. Version: 1.4.

U.S. Food and Drug Administration. (2015 Jul). Food Allergies: What You Need to Know. Retrieved from www.fda.gov/Food/ResourcesForYou/Consumers/ucm079311.htm

INDEX